Program Evaluation
for Exercise Leaders

Program Evaluation for Exercise Leaders

Anita M. Myers, PhD

University of Waterloo
Waterloo, Ontario

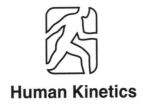

Human Kinetics

Library of Congress Cataloging-in-Publication Data

Myers, Anita M., 1954-
    Program evaluation for exercise leaders / Anita M. Meyers.
      p. cm.
    Includes bibliographical references (p.) and index.
    ISBN 0-88011-709-5
    1. Physical fitness centers--Administration--Evaluation.
  2. Physical education and training--Administration--Evaluation.
  I. Title.
    GV428.5.M49   1999   99-33757
    613.7'068--dc21   CIP

ISBN: 0-88011-709-5

Acquisitions Editors: Michael Bahrke and Becky Lane; **Developmental Editor:** Julie Rhoda; **Assistant Editor:** Sandra Merz Bott; **Copyeditor:** Denelle Eknes; **Proofreader:** Bob Replinger; **Indexer:** Nancy Ball; **Graphic Designer:** Fred Starbird; **Graphic Artist:** Dody Bullerman; **Cover Designer:** Jack W. Davis; **Cartoons:** Tim Offenstein; **Mac Illustrations:** Sharon Smith; **Printer:** Versa Press

Printed in the United States of America   10 9 8 7 6 5 4 3 2 1

Human Kinetics
Web site: http://www.humankinetics.com/

United States: Human Kinetics
P.O. Box 5076
Champaign, IL 61825-5076
1-800-747-4457
e-mail: humank@hkusa.com

Canada: Human Kinetics
475 Devonshire Road Unit 100
Windsor, ON N8Y 2L5
1-800-465-7301 (in Canada only)
e-mail: humank@hkcanada.com

Europe: Human Kinetics, P.O. Box IW14
Leeds LS16 6TR, United Kingdom
+44 (0)113-278 1708
e-mail: humank@hkeurope.com

Australia: Human Kinetics
57A Price Avenue
Lower Mitcham, South Australia 5062
(08) 82771555
e-mail: humank@hkaustralia.com

New Zealand: Human Kinetics
P.O. Box 105-231, Auckland Central
09-523-3462
e-mail: humank@hknewz.com

To the memory of my loving and supportive parents, Ann and John Myers, who taught me that anything is possible if one believes.

Contents

Part I   Why Evaluate Exercise Programs?   1

Chapter 1 Making the Case for Evaluation   3

Chapter 2 Tailoring Recruitment and Delivery Strategies   15

Chapter 3 Customizing Your Client-Information Systems   29

Chapter 7 Interpreting and Using Evaluation Information   *115*

Tool Kit: Worksheet Finder

Foreword

My first job out of school was as a fitness program director for the local family YMCA. I had majored in physical education and paid my tuition by teaching fitness classes along the way. This was the bulk of experience I brought with me to the job at hand.

I paid surprise visits to observe the classes and provide feedback to the instructors on their compliance to class guidelines. Our staff also attended planning retreats. By the end of a grueling weekend, we came up with ideas for promoting and scheduling classes for the upcoming quarter. Some ideas went the way of the dinosaur before the next retreat; others just came up again at the following retreat.

In retrospect, the extent of our evaluation activities consisted of counting the number of people in each class and distributing feedback sheets to those who showed up on the last day of class. Ten people at a 6 A.M. class was seen as OK, but the same number at 5 P.M. was the kiss of death for a fitness class; the quotas seemed arbitrary. Usually, when we scanned the limited remarks on the feedback sheets, there seemed to be more comments about the room temperature than anything else.

One day, my supervisor produced a brief document from the national YMCA describing how to write program goal and objective statements. Suddenly, this was what we had to do for every program. The approach we took was to write objectives, such as to provide instruction, to have three tournaments during the program, or to give certificates of attendance. I'm not sure, however, that anyone ever read the book of goal statements I worked so hard to produce.

After receiving a graduate degree in kinesiology, I went to work for the Centre for Activity and Ageing to develop model exercise programs for older adults—programs that were not only effective but also practical and that the community could implement. I was aware that I would have to do more than head counts. I needed to collect information on what worked and what did not work for each pilot program and make recommendations on how to modify instructor training and delivery. I soon realized that, unlike my graduate thesis research, we could not impose the same stringent controls on real-world program deliverers and participants.

One initiative the Centre for Activity and Ageing was considering was exercise programming and staff training for nursing homes. Before we developed training and programming, it seemed sensible to survey nursing homes in our region to determine the nature of existing exercise programs for residents. We did not want to reinvent the wheel, wasting time and energy. I later realized that what we were doing in collecting this information was a needs assessment.

Concurrently, I worked as an instructor coordinator for a women-only fitness club. I was in charge of scheduling, training, and motivating talented and dedicated fitness instructors, as well as making the necessary decisions to sustain successful fitness classes within a club environment.

My need to learn more about program evaluation was pressing for both my jobs. Luckily, around this time, I heard about a one-day workshop being conducted for health administrators and service deliverers in our area. I, along with the Centre for Activity and Ageing director, quickly signed up.

The workshop was like a ray of light. All the sensible approaches to program planning and development were presented in the context of program evaluation. The workshop facilitator, Anita Myers, applied program evaluation to fitness programs, and we were all glued to our seats. She took the mystery out of terms that before had sounded like Martian. She hit the mark on issues we had been facing but were unsure how to address. She showed us a systematic way of collecting information and how such information could assist us with program decision making. She also showed us how we could cut down paperwork by discarding information we never used.

I was excited that, through program evaluation, I would be able to look a board member in the eye and justify a program. Most important, I could tell paying clients what outcomes they could reasonably expect from participation.

After the workshop, we approached Anita and asked her to assist the Centre for Activity and Ageing with evaluating our training and programming models. Thus began our collaborative relationship. Together, we planned evaluation strategies and developed tools to assess participants. Now, as I've returned to the university, I've had the chance to work with Anita

as my supervisor. I wanted to enhance my skills as a program developer and evaluator and learn more about qualitative techniques, such as focus groups and interviewing.

Today, I'm a practicing program evaluator. I often go back to my workshop and course notes when embarking on a new evaluation project. Currently, I am applying these skills in developing and evaluating a model daily activity program for individuals with chronic illnesses, such as diabetes and osteoporosis, that will be practical and cost-effective.

I confidently endorse the utility of this resource for exercise deliverers and managers. Many examples are based on experiences in fitness programming that we have had over the years. The practical approach to evaluation training Anita uses in her workshops is also evident in this user-friendly book. I only wish that such a book were available to me years ago.

Catrine Tudor-Locke

Preface

Program evaluation is the process of collecting and using information to guide decision making. Evaluation can tell you which aspects of your program are working well and which aspects may need improvement. Evaluation information can guide you in developing cost-effective recruitment, delivery, and retention strategies, tailored to meet client expectations and to maximize participation benefits. Evaluation helps you make confident program decisions based on systematically collected information rather than guesstimates.

This book provides a user-friendly resource on program evaluation written specifically for exercise leaders—both direct service providers and program managers. There are many existing textbooks on program evaluation; however, they tend to be highly technical. Numerous books are available on strategies for developing, marketing, managing, and delivering exercise and activity programs. This is the first book that shows exercise leaders, step-by-step, how to evaluate the development, marketing, and delivery of their own programs.

Program Evaluation for Exercise Leaders explains evaluation approaches in a practical, nontechnical manner and highlights real programs to illustrate the practical utility of evaluation for all types of exercise and activity programming. Exercises at the end of the chapters lead you through the evaluation process, from identifying your own information needs, to collecting the right information for your specific program, to using the information to guide program development and modification. A unique feature of this book is the worksheets developed specifically for exercise programs in collaboration with exercise deliverers. This book illustrates how to use and adapt these features to evaluate your programs.

Part I makes the case for why you should consider program evaluation, whether you work or intend to work in the fitness or health club sector, the corporate sector, the clinical sector, the community sector, the public health sector, or as an independent entrepreneur. In today's competitive fitness market, commercial facilities and personal trainers must position themselves or find their niche in the market place. Nonprofit exercise programs similarly want to attract and keep clients, deliver high-quality services that meet client expectations, maximize client benefits, and minimize adverse effects such as injuries. Evaluation shows you how well you are doing in each area and provides direction for improving your services.

Regardless of which sector of the fitness industry you work in, evaluation can provide the information you need to make routine decisions, such as whether to change class times, hire more staff, or purchase more equipment. Evaluation can also provide the information you need to make long-range planning decisions, such as whether to offer new programs or expand existing services. Equally important, evaluation can provide the evidence you may need to justify your program to others when making the case for a new service, arguing for expansion, or lobbying for additional resources.

Chapter 1 presents nine scenarios, which illustrate that program evaluation can be useful for all programs, regardless of type of exercise or activity, delivery, setting, or clientele. The sources of these scenarios, and other examples used throughout the book, range from large fitness clubs, YMCAs, work sites, and small community programs to the services of self-employed personal trainers. The scenarios also deal with a variety of client groups, ranging from younger to older adults, and from the general public to special groups, such as injured workers, people with diabetes, and nursing home residents.

Chapter 2 addresses the challenges all exercise leaders face in attracting, keeping, and motivating clients. It is important to be aware of different marketing strategies, as well as patterns and projections of exercise participation in various sectors of the fitness industry. Evaluating your programs, however, is necessary to determine whether you are attracting your intended target audience, how your clients compare with similar sectors of the industry, and whether your client profile changes over time. It is also important to be aware of factors that influence program adoption and retention. Evaluation helps you determine how well you are meeting these challenges and ways to improve.

Chapter 3 examines the types of information many programs have at their disposal and shows you how to make better use of this information. Most programs do head counts, but do not systematically track patterns of usage, growth, and attrition. Most instructors know a great deal about individual clients, but do not document the extent of improvement over time and across clients. This book shows you how to customize your record-keeping system to obtain a detailed client profile, to track user and dropout rates, and to document the range and extent of client improvement.

These days, most programs routinely conduct client-satisfaction surveys. However, do you know that most surveys find high rates of satisfaction regardless of whether consumers are purchasing fast foods or exercise services? One reason such surveys tend to be biased is that people who are dissatisfied do not stick around to complete your program-end or year-end survey. You need to be aware of this and other limitations inherent in client-satisfaction surveys and consider other strategies for obtaining feedback from current and former clients.

Part II of this book explains the different approaches to program evaluation—needs assessment, formative, implementation, process, outcome, and cost evaluation. Chapter 4 helps you select the approach that is best suited to your program's objectives, stage of development, and needs for information. Chapter 5 shows you the pros and cons of various ways of collecting information—questionnaires; interviews; focus groups; and fitness, performance, and self-report measures. Practical guidelines help you choose strategies that provide credible information yet do not require extensive resources or training, or overburden your clients.

Part III helps you get started on evaluation. Chapter 6 provides tools for obtaining client consent, collecting background and follow-up information, contacting absent clients, and assessing client change. Because focus groups are one of the best strategies for obtaining in-depth feedback from current clients and potential consumers, I walk you through each step in conducting focus groups. Chapter 7 shows you how to manage and analyze this information manually and using computer software packages. Finally, the book shows you how to interpret, document, and present evaluation findings and recommendations, using written reports and oral presentations with graphics tailored to various audiences.

Although I refer you to additional sources of information, this book is designed as a self-contained resource for busy people who need clear and easy to follow guidelines, but don't have the time to look in a lot of different sources. This book enables you to do your own evaluation with available resources. You can use it to train students, staff, and volunteers, and you can share it with your colleagues. *Program Evaluation for Exercise Leaders* will guide you as you undertake each evaluation activity and discover the benefits of informed decision making.

Acknowledgments

Several groups and individuals contributed to the development of this book. The Canadian Fitness and Lifestyle Research Institute, Fitness Canada, and the Active Living Coalition for Older Adults supported the development of an evaluation framework that laid the groundwork for the present book. The team from the Canadian Centre for Activity and Ageing at the University of Western Ontario, led by Nancy Ecclestone and Don Paterson, provided numerous collaborative opportunities for developing and evaluating leadership training, program delivery, and assessment prototypes. Nancy, Don, Catrine, Darien, Gareth, Shanthi, Clara, Liz, and Rob, I thank you for sharing your wealth of experience with me, and through this book, with colleagues in the field. Catrine Tudor-Locke deserves special mention for her assistance through many brainstorming sessions, feedback on earlier drafts, and always bringing me back to the realities in the field.

Sandy O'Brien Cousins shared her own experiences, encouraged me, and helped me pilot many of the prototype tools. I am also indebted to many other exercise instructors and their participants who used the tools and provided extensive feedback for improvement.

My chairperson, Pat Wainwright, gave me the time I needed to write this book. My friends, particularly Nellie, and my platform tennis team—Judith, Marge, and Rachel—gave me the support and exercise outlets to keep my sanity and my sense of humor, as did my golf partner, Pat Dacey, who also took the time to draft the cartoon concepts.

Finally, I would like to thank Michael Bahrke and all the staff at Human Kinetics for their technical assistance, guidance, and support in seeing this book to completion. My developmental editor, Julie Rhoda, deserves special mention for her insightful suggestions, patience, and prompt feedback to my endless queries.

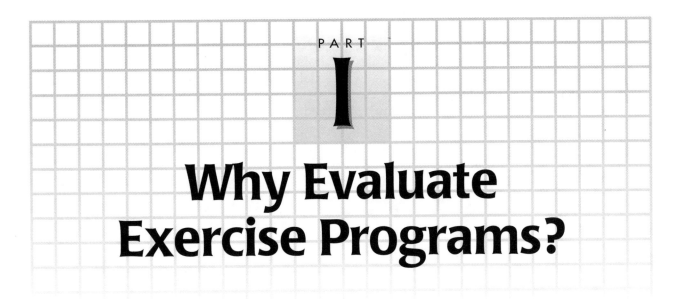

Why Evaluate
Exercise Programs?

Chapter 1 makes the case for why exercise leaders, regardless of type of exercise or activity programming, can benefit from doing program evaluation. The term *exercise leader* is used broadly in this book to encompass the full spectrum of fitness, health promotion, recreation, and clinical providers, and managers of exercise and activity programs and services. As an exercise leader, you may be responsible for only one program or for several programs. Exercise programming and delivery may be your primary duties or only some of your many responsibilities. You may be employed by a commercial facility, a community recreation or public health agency, or a medical clinic. You may be an independent entrepreneur, such as a personal trainer, or you may be a volunteer.

Chapter 1 presents nine scenarios of real programs to illustrate the utility of program evaluation for all types of exercise and all types of leaders. Exercise leaders need information about their clients and their programs to take the guesswork out of decision making. Exercise leaders who operate their own businesses or offer a small community program may be responsible only to their clients and themselves. Most exercise leaders, however, are responsible to other stakeholders in their organization. Some exercise leaders may also be accountable to external stakeholders, such as funders or accreditation bodies. Evaluation provides the evidence you need if you must justify your programs to others.

Chapter 2 addresses challenges inherent in recruiting and retaining clients in all sectors of the fitness industry. Marketing strategies based on principles of affordability, accessibility, and appeal can help you tailor your exercise programs and services to specific target groups. It is important to be aware of trends and projections in the fitness industry. Evaluation is necessary to examine how your clients compare with consumer profiles in similar sectors and whether your client profile changes over time. It is similarly important to be aware of factors that influence exercise adoption and adherence, including recruitment strategies, facility and program features, consumer attitudes and expectations, and motivational techniques. Evaluation is necessary to determine how well you are doing in meeting the expectations of your clientele.

Most programs routinely collect information, often far more information than they use. Chapter 3 looks at the most typical types of information exercise programs have at their disposal and how you can improve record-keeping systems to enhance decision making. Keeping track of your clients allows you to determine patterns in membership growth and attrition. Individual versus aggregate attendance records allow you to determine usage patterns and relate client improvements to participation rate. Examining fitness and other outcomes over time and across clients allows you to determine the extent to which your program is beneficial overall. Although client-satisfaction surveys are popular, you need to be aware of their limitations and consider additional strategies for obtaining feedback from potential, current, and former clients. This book helps you customize your client-information system to collect only the information you want and need to make timely decisions.

Making the Case for Evaluation

1

As an exercise leader, you have likely asked yourself one or more of the following types of questions:

We had a big promotion for our new aquatics class. Why didn't this class fill up?

How can I get more physicians' referrals?

Why are the step classes full but no one comes to the slide classes?

Our surveys suggest that our participants love the program. So why is attendance dropping?

Should we be basing class scheduling and staffing on seasonal attendance rates?

Are phone calls to absentees an efficient use of staff time?

What are peak use periods for the pool? Do certain members use the pool at certain times?

Why are our clients following the diet regimen but not the exercise regimen?

We received a complaint about the music in the weight room. Is this an isolated complaint?

Can we claim that if you join our program you can realistically expect to lose weight?

How do we show the accreditors that injured workers improve in our clinic?

Should part of next year's budget go toward improving the pool or buying weight equipment?

This list of questions could go on and on. The point is that all exercise leaders have questions about their programs or services. Programs constantly make day-to-day and periodic decisions about program promotion, staffing, and delivery, as well as long-range decisions, such as how best to spend next year's budget.

The fitness industry consists of many sectors and types of fitness leaders. For instance, in *Health Fitness Management*, Grantham and colleagues (1998) divide the industry into four broad areas: commercial health clubs and fitness facilities (including single-purpose and multipurpose facilities); community or nonprofit centers (including YMCAs, parks and recreation, country clubs, hotel fitness facilities, residential developments, schools); corporate or work site fitness centers; and clinical programs (including sports medicine, cardiac rehabilitation, physical therapy). Grantham et al. contrasts these four areas with respect to their profit orientation and their relative emphasis on promotion (attracting new members).

These distinctions are not always clear-cut. For instance, hotels, residential developments, work sites, and clinical programs often contract exercise specialists and personal trainers. Thus, the nonprofit sector must also be business conscious and spend their budget wisely. Similarly, there is competition not only in the commercial sector, but also in the clinical sector (for referrals and third-party insurers), the community recreation sector (for tax subsidies), and the public health sector (for government program funding). Regardless of whether exercise facilities and practitioners are looking to make a huge profit on their capital investment, a modest return, or simply to operate on a cost-recovery basis, they still must be consumer focused.

3

Consumers deserve good value for their dollar, whether paying for the exercise service directly or indirectly. Consumers face initiation fees, annual dues, pay-as-you-go plans, fees embedded in hotel charges or condo fees, or fees charged indirectly through taxes—nothing is free!

All exercise and activity programs, services, and facilities have similar objectives:

1. To attract and keep clients
2. To deliver high-quality service
3. To meet clients' needs and expectations
4. To produce positive client outcomes and minimize adverse effects

First and foremost, programs must be accountable to the direct recipients or users of their services. In addition, programs must consider other stakeholder groups, such as indirect recipients, administrators, boards of directors, and funding or accreditation bodies. A *stakeholder* is any individual or group who has a vested interest in the program.

Getting to Know Your Stakeholders

This book will use the term *clients* or *clientele* to refer to direct recipients or consumers of exercise programs, services, and facilities. When discussing particular types of services, I may adapt the lingo. For instance, I may use members of fitness clubs or YMCAs, participants of community programs, patients in cardiac rehabilitation, residents of retirement homes, or employees in work site programs interchangeably with clients.

Direct Recipients

Clients have a right to expect a safe and beneficial program or service, tailored to their needs and expectations, regardless of how much they are paying for the service. Consumers of fitness services are becoming more informed and discriminating. Chapter 2 examines in detail what

consumers look for in a fitness facility or exercise program.

When potential consumers—referrals or guests visiting your facility—ask which program or equipment is best for them, and what benefits they can expect from different program options, can you confidently provide this information? For instance, they may ask you, "How much weight can I expect to lose in six months with this program?" "Will this class help my arthritic pain?" "When will I be able to return to work? How much rehab will I need?"

Many fitness leaders set individual goals, with the client, to tailor the exercise regimen to each client's abilities and expectations. Program evaluation helps you examine the extent of progress across your clientele and over time to determine the proportion who are improving and their range and rate of improvement. Feedback on progress (relative to baseline levels but also relative to other clientele) can be highly motivating to sustain participation. Also, such information can be invaluable for program promotion, as illustrated by a weight-loss clinic flyer: Our clients lose at least 10 pounds in the first month, money-back guarantee.

Indirect Recipients

If your exercise program is directed at clients with special needs—people with injuries, disabilities, or chronic diseases—family members have an important stake in your program. In fact, many programs, such as cardiac rehab programs, encourage spouse or partner participation in the program itself. Family members might ask, "How long will it take (for their family member to return to work or get his or her diabetes under control)?"

Other possible stakeholders are employers and allied health professionals. Employers will ask, "How long will he be off work?" and "Will he need modified duties or special work stations?" Physicians may ask, "Why should I refer my patients to your program?" "What are the benefits that they can realistically expect?" "Will exercise exacerbate their conditions?"

It depends on your exercise service whether you need to be accountable to clients' family members, their employers, or allied health professionals. Figure 1.1 illustrates the possible stakeholder groups of exercise programs and services.

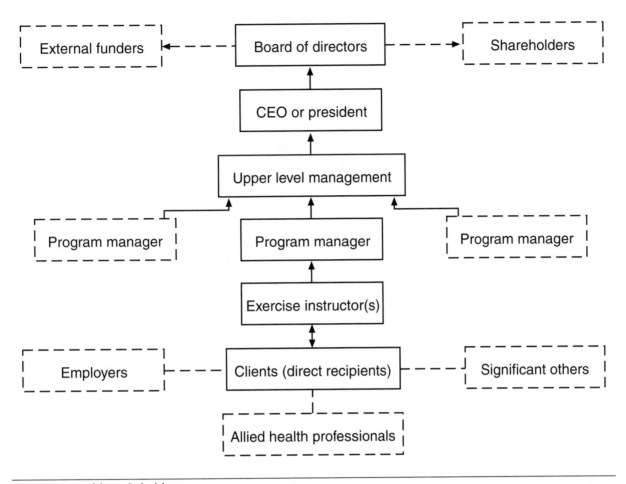

Figure 1.1 Possible stakeholder groups.

Administrators

Unless they are independent entrepreneurs, exercise deliverers usually report to managers. The manager or administrator responsible for a program needs to know the optimum staff- or volunteer-to-client ratio, level of service delivery, and level of program or facility usage to make budgeting and staffing decisions. If funding is cut, administrators need to know which areas they can target without compromising the quality of service delivery. Conversely, if funding is expanded, administrators need to make decisions about whether to allocate additional resources to existing programs or to new initiatives. Administrators can make these decisions more confidently if they have information to answer the following general questions: *What is the current level of staffing (full and part time) relative to program usage? How costly is the program relative to*

usage level and demonstrated participant benefits? More specific examples may be, How much of the time is the pool being used to capacity? Should money go toward improving the pool or buying new resistance equipment—how much is each being used?

Upper level administrators, responsible for multiple programs, will ask, "How do the programs compare in terms of resource allocation, usage, and relative cost-effectiveness?" This stakeholder group frequently reports to a head administrator (agency director, CEO, or president), who, in turn, reports to a board of directors. As Grantham et al. (1998) note, if the CEO is a fitness enthusiast, programs may only need to show evidence concerning membership stability; the benefits of fitness participation are taken for granted. However, today's CEO could be easily replaced by another CEO who will want hard data (beyond bean counting) to support one program over another.

Understanding Lines of Accountability

Lines of accountability are different for commercial and nonprofit exercise programs. Typically, commercial facilities are accountable to boards of directors and sometimes shareholders. Larger nonprofit agencies may also have boards of directors. In addition, nonprofit programs are responsible to external funders, usually local, state, or provincial governments that provide subsidies or tax exemptions. Policy makers, in turn, are ultimately responsible (or should be) to the taxpaying public. These stakeholder groups may decide, for political or personal reasons, that the organization in question should change its priorities. For instance, they may decide to fund more programs for persons with disabilities over the upcoming year.

Believing in your program is important, but may not always be enough. Other parties may challenge your program based on their opinions and agendas. Sitting around a table arguing on the basis of only beliefs and impressions is *not* informed decision making. The people with more clout will usually win the argument. Backing up your arguments with credible information will permit you to argue from a position of strength if you have to justify a new program, lobby for program continuation, or argue for additional funding.

If your agency is subject to external accreditation, as most clinically based programs are, this is definitely a call to action for evaluating your programs. As noted, stakeholders internal to your organization may also request information about your program. Regardless, all managers and front-line service providers should ask themselves the following:

- Is the program meeting the needs and expectations of our clients?
- Who is using our program and to what extent?
- Who is dropping out and why?
- Who is benefiting from our program (increasing fitness, losing weight, etc.)?
- Are there any adverse effects of participation such as injuries?

Program evaluation can provide the information to answer the questions of different stakeholder groups. Simply being told that program evaluation is important, however, is not convincing. You are unlikely to start doing evaluation unless you see it as personally relevant and directly useful to your programs. The next section presents several scenarios that illustrate how information derived through program evaluation can address the challenges exercise deliverers face.

Learning Through Scenarios

The following scenarios reflect the diversity of exercise programming. There are examples from the corporate sector, the commercial sector, the clinical sector, and the community sector. I refer to these scenarios throughout the book to illustrate the practical application of program evaluation. Think about your experiences and questions as you read about the challenges facing the exercise leaders in each scenario.

Scenario 1

Corporate Fitness Program

In your role as director of occupational health and safety, you decide to offer an on-site exercise program for the 100 employees at your computer software design company. Your objectives are to foster the image that your company cares about its employees, to increase the fitness level of your office workers, to reduce work-related injuries, and to reduce absenteeism. You have read the results of a large trial conducted with employees of the Johnson & Johnson Co. (Jones et al. 1990), which found reduced absenteeism in sites that offered a fitness class.

You hire a certified fitness instructor who suggests basing the program on the guidelines by the American College of Sports Medicine (ACSM 1995). With the instructor, you decide to offer the exercise class Mondays, Wednesdays, and Fridays after usual office hours (from 4:30 to 5:30 P.M.). The class will be held on site in the workout studio built by the company a few years ago. The program will include warm-up and cool-down periods, with 40 minutes of moderate- to high-intensity aerobic exercises at 60 percent to 90 percent of maximum age-predicted heart rate. Participants will be taught to monitor their heart rates.

After a few months, you ask your instructor, "How's it going? Do they like it?" As you requested, she administered a satisfaction questionnaire at the end of the first month. The 15 people who filled out the survey gave high ratings to the class and the instructor. You were pleased by these results. However, you are concerned when the instructor reports that the average class attendance has dropped from 20 people at the beginning to fewer than 10 now.

You ask yourself, "Why did only 20 percent of our employees try this class? Why did some people stop coming? What is it about the 10 people who kept coming?" Chapter 4 illustrates that you can address questions concerning usage patterns, and comparisons of continuing versus discontinuing clients, through process evaluation.

Scenario 2
Textile Plant Wellness Program

You are a health educator employed by a regional public health unit. The health statistics for your region indicate that obesity and smoking are prevalent. A recent telephone survey indicated that many adults do not exercise regularly (defined on the survey as three times a week for at least 30 minutes). Favorite leisure activities for adult males in the region consist of fishing and hunting. For adult females, watching television ranked as the most popular. The demographic profile for the region indicates predominately young adults with families. You decide to begin health promotion activities by targeting the textile plant that is the major employer for the region. This work site consists of primarily blue-collar employees, many of whom are women. You have in mind a program for women that would emphasize weight loss, nutrition, and exercise. You have even thought of a possible name: Time for Me.

You ask yourself, "Will these women be interested in such a program? How should we offer the program, where, and when?" As chapter 4 discusses, you can address these types of questions through needs assessment, which examines the views of the intended target audience. If the findings of the needs assessment provide support for the program, formative evaluation would be useful to pilot test the program name, recruitment strategies, and draft program materials. This in-

formation helps you decide whether to proceed with program implementation.

Scenario 3
Tai Chi Program at a YMCA

As a YMCA manager, you are reading the latest batch of member comments from the suggestion box. Several people suggest you offer a Tai Chi program. One person even dropped in a newspaper clipping describing the ancient Chinese exercise and extolling the physical (flexibility, coordination, and balance) and mental (relaxation) benefits of Tai Chi. You think that Tai Chi classes may be particularly appealing to your older adult clients, although your Active Older Adult Program area already offers aquatics, dance, and general conditioning programs. You have the YMCA resource manual on older adult programming (Hooke and Zoller 1992) on your shelf, which suggests advantages of both age-integrated and age-segregated programming.

You ask yourself, "Should Tai Chi classes be open to all ages, or should we offer separate classes for older and younger adults?" You want to know whether your membership is interested in such a program. You also wonder whether Tai Chi may draw in new members, perhaps on an a la carte or pay-as-you-go basis. Needs assessment can provide such information.

As you start planning this new program, you become curious about the relative interest levels among your older adult clientele in the existing programming options your YMCA provides. As I show in chapters 2 and 3, tracking participants across programs to determine the extent of concurrent or multiple program participation, as well as the extent to which people switch programs, can be informative in facility-wide planning.

Scenario 4
Active Living Posters and Mall-Walking Program

You are a health educator employed by a public health agency in a northern community. You surf the Internet and see the United States Surgeon General's (United States Department of Health and Human Services 1996) report on physical activity and health, which advocates moderate exercise, such as walking 30 minutes a day, ideally most days of the week. You are also aware of the Canadian Society for Exercise Physiology's (CSEP 1996) *Guide to Healthy Active Living.* These public health messages are something you can work with to promote physical activity in your community.

You decide to develop posters on the benefits of active living, particularly regular walking, and display these posters in the three malls in your community. You recruit volunteers to lead daily walking groups in the three malls from January to March. You will need to decide whether to continue the program into the spring and summer and whether to offer the same program next fall and winter. As chapter 4 shows, several evaluation approaches apply to this scenario. Process evaluation will help you determine usage patterns and examine the effectiveness of your recruitment strategies. Outcome evaluation can help you examine the benefits associated with participation in the mall-walking program.

Scenario 5
Rehabilitation Clinic for Injured Workers

You are the director of a private rehabilitation clinic, with a background in kinesiology. Your clientele are primarily injured workers with musculoskeletal, low-back injuries. Workers' compensation pays for eligible clients to attend. Based on their guidelines, your clinic uses an intensive, individualized exercise conditioning regimen, with education on correct lifting techniques and other strategies to prevent the reoccurrence of back injuries. Your staff includes a physician and a chiropractor, as well as physical, occupational, and massage therapists.

The workers' compensation board requires you to collect and report demographic and diagnostic information on all referrals, as well as a return to work recommendation at discharge. Recently, policy makers at the workers' compensation board have expressed concerns about whether early referral (as soon as possible after the injury) is the best practice. They also recognize that return to work may be influenced by several factors: job satisfaction, job demands, employer considerations, and the spontaneous or natural recovery process of low-back pain. Your

funders question how much bang they are receiving for their buck. They ask all their currently accredited rehabilitation clinics, including yours, to provide additional indicators of client recovery over the next six months.

Chapter 4 helps you develop performance indicators and targets, and link these to various program components. Chapter 5 helps you select the best tools for measuring desired client outcomes, in this case, client recovery.

Scenario 6
Exercise Programming in a Nursing Home

You have recently been hired as a part-time recreation director in a nursing home. You are a certified fitness instructor. You have taken specialized training for working with older adults and have read Spirduso's (1995) *Physical Dimensions of Aging*, as well as Van Norman's (1995) *Exercise Programming for Older Adults*. However, your work experience to date has been with healthy, community-living seniors. Your observation of the nursing home is that most residents spend a large proportion of the time lying or sitting. Many people are wheeled to and from the dining room and the activities. The existing exercise program run by your predecessor is chair based, consisting of simple, range-of-motion exercises to music.

At a recent conference for people working in the area of physical activity and aging, you saw an innovative model presented by a group from Canada (Lazowski et al. 1997). They showed that a challenging exercise program was not only feasible, but more beneficial than the usual seated programs for nursing home residents. Similarly, you plan to train staff and volunteers concerning the benefits of mobilization, strength, and balance training. In addition to a new exercise class, you would like to get a walking program going in the home.

You meet with the head administrator and medical director to discuss your exciting ideas. They respond, "Anything that keeps them busy is OK, so long as it is not too strenuous and does not agitate them. Go ahead and try it, as long as it does not cost too much."

You have already started doing evaluation by observing the status quo—the general level of resident mobility and the existing exercise class. Your motivation for more formally evaluating your initiatives is to demonstrate to the head administrator and medical director that more challenging exercise programming for the residents is not only feasible, but can have therapeutic benefits. You want to confront existing attitudes about the capabilities of these frail residents and the value of exercise as "just another activity."

Scenario 7
Diabetes Self-Management Program

One of your responsibilities is to oversee a group-based education program delivered by diabetes educators to assist persons newly diagnosed with Type 2 diabetes in managing their condition. The three-day program covers the following topics: complications of diabetes, oral medications and insulin, dietary modifications, weight control, blood glucose monitoring, foot care, and physical activity. Patients are encouraged to bring a family member. All workshop attendees are given a take-home booklet summarizing the content of the educational sessions. You are concerned that current guidelines concerning exercise are vague.

You want to know, "What messages on exercise are the diabetes educators conveying? How are clients perceiving the message? What messages are these people with Type 2 diabetes getting from other health professionals involved in their care? What were the physical activity practices of these clients before coming to the clinic, and do their practices change as a result of the educational program?"

This program is interested in scrutinizing its existing curriculum or program content concerning one component, physical activity. By examining what they are actually delivering (through process evaluation), and what impacts, if any, the current program is having on clients (through outcome evaluation), the program can decide whether to modify the curriculum. Chapter 4 outlines the steps involved in process and outcome evaluation, and chapter 5 provides options for collecting information to address the questions of this coordinator.

Scenario 8
Community Wellness Clinics

As director of a senior's center, you have developed a peer-led program (called 55 Alive and Well). The program aims to provide current information on healthy lifestyles and to enable older adults to attain and maintain their optimal level of physical, mental, emotional, and social functioning. The program consists of a once a week exercise class (led by a senior who has taken a fitness instructor leadership course), followed by a guest speaker. Weekly topics include nutrition, medication use, stress management, fall prevention, driving, care giving, and so on.

To see how well you are doing, you develop and distribute a satisfaction questionnaire at the end of each session for four consecutive weeks. You are not sure what to do with all the forms you have collected. This book will help you aggregate and interpret this information. After reading chapter 3, however, you may reconsider using client-satisfaction surveys as the only approach to evaluating your program.

Scenario 9
Personal Training

You have a university degree in physical education and tried teaching high school for a few years. That wasn't for you, and you decided to become a personal trainer. You now hold professional certification for personal trainers, as well as being certified as a massage therapist. You are ready to open your own business. You plan to offer fitness appraisals, exercise prescription with supervised sessions, massage therapy, and stress and weight management. Your university buddy, now a family physician, says he will refer his patients to you and prescreen for undiagnosed heart conditions and other contraindications. You talk things over and decide you will go after the niche market of persons aged 40 to 69.

You are debating whether to offer your services out of your home gym, out of a mobile van, or at the workplaces or homes of your clientele. You plan to keep track of how many clients come from your physician contact, your newspaper ads, and word-of-mouth referrals from satisfied customers.

You would like to document improvement rates in fitness, weight, and stress across your clientele for ammunition when approaching other physicians for referrals. In other words, you plan to evaluate your efforts. This book will show you how.

The above scenarios illustrate that program evaluation is useful for, and can be applied to, all programs—regardless of type of exercise, type of delivery, setting, or target group. Programs come in all shapes and sizes.

A program is any organized or purposeful activity or set of activities delivered to a designated target group. A program can consist of a class, a pamphlet or booklet, a poster, a video, a prescribed regimen, or a combination of interventions.

As noted earlier in the chapter, the sponsorship of the program and whether it is embedded in a larger organization or agency determines the type of stakeholders involved and the information you need for decision making. Some scenarios illustrated demands for external accountability, such as from the workers' compensation board in the case of the rehabilitation clinic. Because this body pays for injured workers to attend the clinics and accredits these clinics, they have the right to request information on program effectiveness.

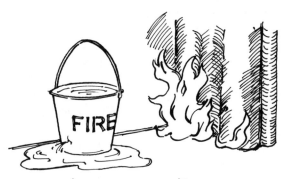

Are you prepared?

In other scenarios, the request for information was internal to the organization. For instance, in the first scenario, the director of occupational health and safety asked the fitness instructor to provide feedback on attendance and participant satisfaction. In the nursing home scenario, the recreational director was not asked to evaluate her new program initiatives. However, she wanted to demonstrate to the head administrator and medical director that challenging programming was feasible and more effective than the exercise class delivered by her predecessor. The most powerful motivator for doing program evaluation is to address your needs for information. For instance, the personal trainer wanting to establish his business was keenly interested in tracking patterns of referral and documenting client improvements to promote his services.

If you are thinking, "Program evaluation sounds exciting, but we do not have the expertise or time to do evaluation," you are not alone. There are several misconceptions about evaluation, particularly concerning technical expertise, additional workload, and fear of negative findings. Let's address and dispel these myths.

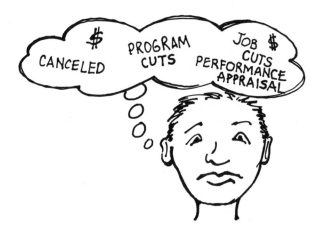

Demystifying Program Evaluation

As this book demonstrates, you can do evaluation even with limited resources and no formal research training. You do not have to be a researcher to evaluate your programs. Table 1.1 illustrates the fundamental differences between research and program evaluation.

Researchers study hypotheses of academic interest, and evaluation examines questions or issues of interest to the program. Regardless of whether program personnel conduct their own data collection or hire external consultants, the

Table 1.1 Key Distinctions Between Research and Program Evaluation

Research	Evaluation
Purpose	
Advances scholarly knowledge Reviewed by peers Is published	Provides information for decision making Answers to stakeholders Has practical utility
Focus	
Examines efficacy under highly controlled, artificial conditions Subjects are carefully selected Has strict inclusion, exclusion criteria	Examines effectiveness and efficiency under real-world conditions or normal operation Participants are self-selected No restrictions
Methods	
Rigorous methodologies Research assistants collect data Batteries of tests Significant group differences	Good enough methodologies Staff and volunteers collect data Practical assessments Relative client benefits (% improving)

purpose is still the same—to provide useful information for program decision making. Research findings are judged by other researchers and disseminated in scholarly journals. Credibility and utility of evaluation findings, meanwhile, are judged by program stakeholders. Oral presentations and discussions among stakeholders about the findings are often more influential than written evaluation reports. Evaluation findings must be timely; that is, they must be available for planning next year's budget and program offerings.

Research examines the *efficacy* of interventions under highly controlled conditions. Single studies often focus on only one type of exercise, such as endurance training, and manipulate one aspect of exercise, such as intensity level. Other aspects, such as frequency and duration, are held constant for the study. Research studies use *subjects* who are carefully selected using strict inclusion and exclusion criteria. Subjects who do not follow the strict study protocol, such as those who do not attend enough sessions or those who start exercising outside, may be dropped from the study. In general, people who are selected for and agree to take part in research studies tend to be educated, literate, healthy, health conscious, motivated, and compliant.

In contrast, evaluation examines the *effectiveness* (client outcomes) and *efficiency* (cost and feasibility) of programs under real-world conditions. Programs are rarely delivered under ideal circumstances with optimal resources. Exercise leaders attempt to deliver the best programs they can with the resources at their disposal. For instance, you may want to deliver a program three times a week but only have the staff or volunteers to offer it once or twice a week.

Evaluation examines program delivery under conditions of routine operation and with self-selected participants. You do not ask people to leave the program because they choose not to attend regularly. Part of your challenge as an instructor is to constantly motivate your clients. Some clients may have health problems, physical disabilities, or cognitive impairments. They may not even be convinced that exercise is for them. You accept these challenges as an exercise leader.

Researchers use rigorous methodologies, such as random selection and randomized designs with control groups, to enhance scientific credibility. Batteries of measures are administered before and after the exercise intervention. Subjects may be dropped from data analyses if they cannot or will not undergo fitness testing or complete questionnaires.

In contrast, evaluation balances credibility with practicality in selecting options for data collection. Programs may not have sophisticated testing equipment or the expertise to use such equipment. Staff or volunteers, rather than highly trained research assistants, often must collect evaluation information. Practical considerations—ease of administering, scoring, and interpreting—become as important as the reliability and validity of the measurement tools. Evaluation also accepts the challenge to obtain feedback from all participants or as many as possible. For instance, if self-report questionnaires are too difficult for participants with poor reading abilities, interviews may be necessary.

The misconception that evaluation requires technical expertise is related to the myth that it requires more work and time. As chapter 3 discusses, you probably already collect at least some client information you need for evaluation. This book helps you customize your information-keeping systems to meet your needs. Evaluation planning may actually decrease the amount of time you and your staff spend on information gathering.

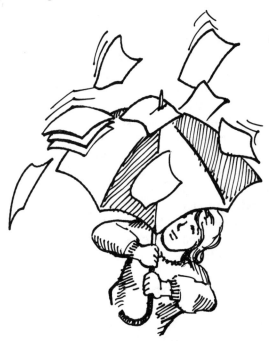

Another source of resistance to program evaluation is the fear of negative findings, which in turn could lead to program cuts and staff layoffs. As chapter 4 shows, it is not productive to think of programs as successes or failures. This way of thinking stems from traditional research in which the aim is to find statistically significant differences between experimental and control groups. In the real world, programs tend to be relatively effective or beneficial—for some clients more than for others. By setting realistic program objectives, your program will be judged against your performance targets. The aim of evaluation is to discover ways to improve your program and maximize client benefits. Rarely are programs cut based on evaluation information; in fact, you can use evaluation results to lobby for additional resources.

Finally, staff and volunteers often worry that their own performance is being judged during program evaluation. Hiring qualified staff, orienting staff and volunteers, and periodically reviewing competencies are important issues in organization management, as is compliance with facility standards (ACSM 1997a; Grantham et al. 1998). To foster buy-in to evaluation, however, it is critical to reassure staff that it is *not* their individual performance, but rather program delivery (including location, content, music, group composition) as a total package that is the objective of evaluation.

> **K**eep program evaluation distinct from staff performance appraisals.

Applying Research and Programming Guidelines

I do not want to leave you with the impression that research has no value for exercise programming. The corporate fitness program described in the first scenario was developed using ACSM (1995) guidelines. Participants were taught to monitor their heart rates to ensure they were following the prescribed intensity for achieving aerobic benefits. Because of decades of research on aerobic training, these data are generalizable; if these employees (young adult males) follow the prescribed program, they can expect to achieve both short-term benefits (enhanced cardiovascular fitness) and long-term benefits (reduced mortality from cardiovascular and other diseases).

There is also substantial research evidence that work site fitness programs can lead to reduced absenteeism (Jones et al. 1990). Given such solid evidence in this area, outcome evaluation may be less important for this program. Process evaluation (explained in chapter 4), however, is necessary to determine why only 20 percent of the employees were interested in this program and why attendance dropped after a few months.

Based on exercise research to date, we know more about the benefits of high-intensity aerobic exercise than we do about low- and moderate-endurance exercise or about resistance or flexibility regimens. We know more about cardiorespiratory fitness outcomes than about other outcomes of exercise or about process variables (factors affecting recruitment and adherence). We know more about athletes and young males than about other populations, and we know more about prescribing and adherence patterns for postcardiac patients than about groups with other diseases and disabilities. A case in point concerns persons with Type 2 diabetes, for which published, recommended exercise guidelines are not only unclear but contradictory (Tudor-Locke et al. 1998). As noted in *Exercise Management for Persons with Chronic Diseases and Disabilities* (ACSM 1997b), "Many diseases and disabilities have not been sufficiently studied to yield exact dose-response information, recommendations are vague, coming not from controlled trials but from empiricism and anecdote" (p. 3).

The active living posters and mall-walking program depicted in the fourth scenario were based on the public health recommendation put forth by a panel of experts (Pate et al. 1995), and subsequently endorsed by the U.S. Surgeon General (United States Department of Health and Human Services 1996). This group of experts agreed that the scientific evidence was sufficient to argue that regular, moderate-intensity physical activity—equivalent to 30 minutes or two miles of brisk walking—confers substantial health benefits.

Keep in mind that the preceding recommendation still focuses on the role of endurance exercise for general health benefits. It is recognized that other fitness components—muscle strength and flexibility—should not be overlooked, particularly for older adults (Pate et al. 1995; United States Department of Health and Human Services 1996). The World Health Organization (WHO 1997) has recently issued guidelines for promoting physical activity among older persons. Scientific evidence for the benefits of strength training, flexibility training, and balance training concerning various populations is emerging. Also, researchers are now examining not only the fitness benefits, such as cardiorespiratory fitness and muscle strength, but also the functional, psychological, and social benefits of exercise participation.

Students in exercise physiology, kinesiology, physical education, and health studies programs are exposed to the latest research articles and textbooks summarizing scientific research in the exercise field. There are now courses on special populations, such as persons with disabilities or older adults. Increasingly, academic departments are also offering courses on program development, marketing, and evaluation.

Once out of school, however, exercise leaders often do not have the time to keep up with the volume of scientific journals and academic textbooks published in the exercise field. Review papers and consensus reports are easier to access, especially if you use the Internet. Such papers and reports tend to be far less technical than research articles and quickly deliver the bottom line. Periodic position papers show how the field is changing. For instance, in 1978, the ACSM position paper on the recommended quantity and quality of exercise for healthy adults focused solely on cardiorespiratory fitness and body composition. By 1990, the ACSM included recommendations on resistance training. By 1998, the ACSM included flexibility exercises and the health benefits of low-intensity exercise (ACSM 1998a). A separate position paper concerning exercise for older adults has also been released by the ACSM (1998b). Position statements are emerging for particular disease groups, such as the 1997 paper on exercise and diabetes put out by the ACSM and the American Diabetes Association. It is worthwhile for all exercise leaders to keep up with these position statements.

Fortunately, several books are now available that provide straightforward, practical guidelines for the promotion and marketing, development, delivery, and management of exercise programs and facilities (e.g., Cotton, Ekeroth, and Yancy 1998; Grantham et al. 1998; Miller 1995; Van Norman 1995). However, guidelines are just that—guidelines. You still need to examine the results of your advertising strategies. You still need to identify the benefits you can reasonably expect from your program and examine the extent to which your participants are achieving such benefits. Many exercise programming books stress the importance of program evaluation. This book shows you how to do evaluation in a systematic yet practical manner.

Summary

Some programs require information for accountability purposes—to justify developing new programs or to argue for continued or additional funding for existing programs. All programs require information for internal planning and day-to-day decision making. I used nine scenarios to illustrate that program evaluation applies to all programs regardless of size, type of exercise, mode of delivery, setting, or clientele. You do not have to be a researcher to evaluate your programs.

Programs can look to the research literature for models of delivery, potential outcomes, and standardized measurement tools. However, programmers cannot wait for conclusive research findings to be published. Even programs modeled after research studies are rarely implemented as planned. We need to be cautious in generalizing research findings, because studies differ from programs and subjects differ from participants.

Practical guidelines developed by experienced practitioners are also available for suggestions

on promotion, programming, and testing. However, most programs make modifications to suit their particular settings, participants, and available resources. Even if you follow programmatic guidelines closely, you still need to evaluate your recruitment and delivery efforts and the extent to which your clients benefit from participation.

Working Exercises

To apply the concepts from this chapter to your program, either try these exercises yourself or with other exercise leaders involved in your program. If you are responsible for more than one program, do each program separately.

1. Make a list of questions—what you would like to know—about your program and your participants. How might such information help you to make decisions about modifying current recruitment, targeting, or delivery efforts? (Look back at the scenarios for examples.)

2. Identify the stakeholders of your program. List the types of things each stakeholder group might want to know about the program. (Look back at the section on stakeholders.)

3. Consider the extent to which your program has been modeled after research studies or general programmatic guidelines. In what ways has it been modified or adapted and why?

Tailoring Recruitment and Delivery Strategies

CHAPTER

2

"The fitness revolution that began in the 1970s was aimed primarily at the young and the fit" (Cotton, Ekeroth, and Yancy 1998, xi). Now, on the other hand, experts project that the senior market represents the greatest potential for growth in the fitness industry into the next century. Awareness of exercise consumption patterns and projections is helpful for positioning your services in the marketplace. Collecting your own information, however, is critical to identify the potential market in your area, examine whether you are reaching your intended audience, compare your client profile to similar sectors of the fitness industry, and determine whether your client profile is changing over time.

This chapter addresses the challenges many exercise leaders face in attracting, keeping, and motivating clients. The first section discusses the strategic targeting of exercise programs and services in today's competitive marketplace. The second section reviews population patterns and projections in exercise participation. The third section discusses challenges in segmenting the market of exercise consumers into distinct groups based on demographic characteristics, abilities, and lifestyles. The last section reviews factors that have been shown to influence program adoption and adherence. Awareness of these factors can assist you in tailoring recruitment and delivery strategies. Evaluation, however, is critical to determine which strategies are most effective and which areas you can modify to better meet the needs and expectations of your clientele.

Targeting Exercise Services

Recall from chapter 1 that the *target audience* is the individuals or groups for which you intend the program or service. Whether you are marketing running shoes, exercise videos, fitness facilities, personal training services, or exercise classes, you can more successfully reach your audience and sell your product by tailoring your promotional and delivery strategies to specific types of consumers, as opposed to using a shotgun approach and trying to appeal to everyone.

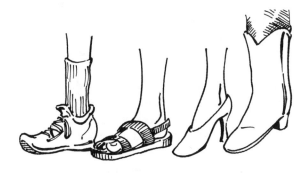

Strategic marketing is the key to successfully promoting all exercise services—programs, facilities, equipment, clothing, and sporting events. The field of social marketing has brought together commercial marketing concepts, social psychological theories of persuasion and communication, and program evaluation strategies (Kotler 1976; Kotler and Anderson 1987). The principles of social marketing have been applied to mass media health education (cf. U.S. Department of

Health and Human Services 1992), to marketing sport products and events (cf. Mullin, Hardy, and Sutton 1993), and to marketing fitness facilities and programs (cf. Grantham et al. 1998).

From a social marketing perspective, exercise services are products that consumers are more likely to purchase if the mix of price (affordability), place (accessibility), and promotion (appeal to interests and preferences) is customized to their needs, expectations, and demands.

Matching service costs to purchasers' income appears straightforward. The most important factor regarding affordability, however, may not be income, but what consumers view as their discretionary income (Grantham et al. 1998). People typically weigh several things when making choices concerning how to spend their leisure time and money, and they make trade-offs. For instance, some people are willing to pay more for exercise options that are located closer to their workplace or home. Others are willing to travel farther to get the services they want. For some, accessibility means proximity in location; others want free parking. Still others are interested in club hours or class scheduling.

One key concept of social marketing is *segmentation*. Segmentation entails dividing the general market into distinct, homogeneous groups of potential buyers.

You can segment potential consumers by demography (i.e., income level, education, age, gender, education, ethnicity); geography (proximity of residence or workplace to the program or facility); psychography (attitudes and lifestyles, i.e., where and how people spend their time); health profiles; fitness profiles; or any combination of these characteristics. The following section reviews patterns and projections of exercise consumption by different population segments.

Population Patterns and Projections

The proportion of North American adults that is physically active has grown from about 10 percent in 1960 to about 50 percent by the mid-1990s. Today, only half the population is considered active enough to derive health benefits from exercise according to the Canadian Fitness and Lifestyles Research Institute (CFLRI 1996a) and the United States Surgeon General (United States Department of Health and Human Services 1996). Inactivity is still more common for women, nonwhites, older adults, and persons with little education and income. These groups constitute the harder-to-reach segments of the population.

Encouraging sedentary adults to lead more active lifestyles by promoting options that do not require athletic skills or user fees is on top of the public health agenda. Organizing equipment exchanges and rentals; partnering with local businesses or service organizations to sponsor teams, pool, or rink use; waiving registration fees for low-income individuals; and promoting public walking and biking trails are strategies for promoting equitable access to physical activity (CFLRI 1996b). The philosophy of some organizations is that no one is turned away for inability to pay (cf. YMCA 1995).

The commercial sector, on the other hand, continues to target primarily the white, middle- and upper-class segments of the population, and more narrowly, the fit, healthy, and younger members of this segment. In Canada, single adults, particularly males, currently spend the most on exercise (CFLRI 1996b). Persons with university educations and higher incomes spend more across all age groups. The largest expenditure is for equipment, followed by user fees, transportation, and instruction. In both Canada and the United States, the retail fitness industry is booming and revenues continue to grow despite a fluctuating economy.

The segment of the North American population that is active tends to use various types of facilities—both commercial and nonprofit—often in addition to exercising in home and work environments (CFLRI 1996c). Home exercise has increased 80 percent between 1987 and 1997. During the same period, there was a 50 percent increase in fitness club participation (Grantham et al. 1998). This translates into a market penetration of 8 percent of the American population (or about 20 million people) participating in some type of health and fitness facility away from home. Currently, multipurpose health and fitness clubs are capturing the largest market share; YMCAs rank second; single-purpose facilities, such as aquatic centers, racket clubs, aerobic studies, rank third; and corporate fitness centers a distant fourth (Grantham et al. 1998).

According to Grantham et al. (1998), trends now evident in the commercial sector are

- movement from single- to multipurpose centers;
- increased popularity of personalized services, such as personal training;
- payment systems that hold clubs accountable to members, such as monthly fees versus annual dues; and
- a shift to comprehensive wellness programming, including massage, nutrition, and mind-body programs, such as Yoga and Tai Chi.

Although new exercise fads, programs, and equipment will continue to emerge, Grantham et al. predict that it is "doubtful that few will take the place of walking, swimming, cardiovascular equipment, weight training, and cycling. These five categories will continue to dominate the interests of mainstream fitness enthusiasts" (1998, 40).

Marketing surveys indicate that today's typical consumer of commercial fitness clubs is between the ages of 18 and 34, has a college degree, and has an annual income over $75,000. In contrast, the typical YMCA member is between 35 and 54 and has an annual income between $25,000 and $49,000. The ratio of males to females is roughly equal in the commercial and nonprofit sectors; though males tend to dominate the corporate fitness sector. Although only 12 percent of commercial club memberships are currently held by seniors, it is noteworthy that this segment uses these facilities more often than any other age group (Grantham et al. 1998).

One important change between the mid-1980s and the mid-1990s is that persons over the age of 55 have increased their exercise participation by 70 percent (Grantham et al. 1998). There has already been a rapid growth in senior fitness certification. The proliferation of books in this area (i.e., Van Norman 1995; Cotton, Ekeroth, and Yancy 1998) attest to the growing interest in programming for this target group. Active Older Adults has become a priority program area for the USA-YMCA (Hooke and Zoller 1992). Due to changing demographics, the fitness industry will increasingly pursue the senior market.

Keeping a close watch on demographic patterns is as important for the fitness industry as for real estate developers, school boards, the cosmetic industry, or health care funders. For instance, in *Boom, Bust, and Echo*, Foot (1996) describes the tennis craze of the 1980s, in which tennis clubs had waiting lists, public courts were crowded, and sporting goods dealers could not keep up with the demand for the latest in shoes and rackets. By the mid-1990s, however, tennis participation was down dramatically, and tennis clubs found themselves advertising for new members. Foot argues that changing demographics were responsible for this phenomenon. The bulk of tennis enthusiasts are young adults, and the boom of the 1980s coincided with the fact that the baby boom cohort, making up about a third of the population, were in their prime tennis-playing years.

Several countries, particularly Canada, the United States, and Australia, experienced a significant baby boom following World War II and lasting until the early 1960s. By comparison, the cohorts born before World War II and right after the boomers (the baby bust cohort) are small. The offspring of the boomers—the baby boom echo (born from 1980 to 1995)—is also a large cohort. Due to sheer numbers, and thus purchasing power, when baby boomers get interested in something for themselves or their children, marketers take notice. For instance, on-site day care centers and supervised programming for their kids are attractive club features for today's busy middle-aged boomer couples in which both parents are working.

The baby boomer bulge will account for a significant proportion of older adults into the next century. This age cohort has driven and will continue to drive the fitness market. In the 1970s and 1980s, baby boomers were in their early adulthood and responsible for market trends such as the tennis boom. By the 1990s, this large age cohort was middle age and their personal fitness needs and interests changed. The current popularity of low-impact classes and golf is largely due to the baby boomers. Baby boomers and their children currently dominate the membership growth in health and fitness facilities. Projections are that by 2010, fitness memberships of the 18 to 34 age group will decline significantly, but the 55 and over group will grow by 13 percent annually (Grantham et al. 1998).

Population aging is occurring worldwide. For instance, by the year 2015, it is projected that 23 percent of Japan's population will be over the age of 65 (Harada 1994). By the year 2021, 20 percent of Canada's population will be over 65. Although the total U.S. population is 10 times larger than

Canada, population-aging trends are similar. In sheer numbers, by 2030, 65.6 million Americans (or 1 in 5) will be over 65 (Ferrini and Ferrini 1993). Due to life expectancy patterns, there will be more older women than older men.

Later in this chapter, we examine the expectations of today's seniors with respect to tailoring exercise programming. Here it is important to note that, in the future, older adults will compose a much larger potential market, and tomorrow's seniors will have different needs and demands. In contrast to current generations of older adults, baby boomers grew up with different physical education curricula, different attitudes, and far more opportunities for sport and leisure skill development. Experts agree that baby boomers will shape the fitness industry over the next few decades (Cotton, Ekeroth, and Yancy 1998; Grantham et al. 1998; Van Norman 1995).

Challenges in Market Segmentation

Market segmentation is most useful if you are considering expanding your client base. Segmenting the market of exercise consumers, however, is not as straightforward as it may appear—even when you consider only one demographic characteristic, such as age. Currently, exercise programming is broadly segmented into youth, adult, and older adult categories. Age 18 is typically used to separate youth from adult programming. Although young and middle-aged adults are likely to be attracted to different types of programming, often these groups are not targeted separately. Recall that the largest segment of the North American population—the baby boomers—are currently in their mid-30s to early 50s.

Age 65 has customarily marked the beginning of retirement. However, due to early retirement patterns, many fitness and wellness older adult programs are now targeting adults 55 and over. Older adults should not be lumped into a single group. For instance, Van Norman (1995) suggests that programming must be tailored differently for seniors who are healthy and fit, for those who are healthy but unfit, and for those who are both unhealthy and unfit. Spirduso (1995), meanwhile, recommends five segments, ranging from the

physically elite to the physically dependent older adult. Both classifications consider physical abilities more important than age per se when it comes to suitable exercise programming for older adults.

You should also consider other criteria, such as gender, in segmenting potential fitness consumers. The preferences of different ethnic groups, such as African Americans and Hispanics in the United States or aboriginal populations in Canada, the United States, or Australia, are also important, but to date have received little attention. The special needs of the disabled and chronically ill are beginning to receive more attention from the clinical sector (cf. Miller 1995), but to date have limited attention from the fitness industry as a whole.

In any case, before going after a new market, you need to find out about the characteristics of the population residing in your *catchment area.* Your catchment area may be defined by city limits, suburbs, or proximity (for instance, people living within a 10-mile radius of your facility). Voter lists or other household lists are a good way to obtain a demographic profile of your area. Local public health boards usually have demographic, health, and social indicator information, such as family composition and income distribution. You do not want to spend time and money developing a whole line of programs for older adults if your area consists primarily of young families. Conversely, you would think twice about providing on-site day care if you learn that your area is dominated by retirees. Also, if your area has a high concentration of certain ethnic groups, you may want to consider promoting your services to these groups.

Feasibility of market segmentation depends on the size of the segment, responsiveness of the segment to the product, and available resources for promotion, packaging, and delivery (Mullin, Hardy, and Sutton 1993). Once you ascertain that a sufficient potential market exists in your area, you still need to gauge the level of interest or responsiveness among these potential consumers. You also need to determine the best way to reach your target audience and whether your recruitment strategies are cost-effective. The next section examines what consumers look for and expect from fitness centers and exercise programs (i.e., what influences people to join various exercise clubs or programs).

Factors Influencing Program Adoption

The three areas that I will discuss in this section are recruitment strategies, facility and program features, and consumer expectations. All three are important considerations in attracting potential consumers. First, the consumer must be aware that your service is available. Second, the consumer must be interested in your service package. Third, your promotion must live up to its promises and the consumer's expectations.

Recruitment Strategies

As a rule, 10 percent of total annual expenses for a start-up organization and 5 percent for a mature organization should go toward increasing their market share or recruiting new clients (Mullin, Hardy, and Sutton 1993). Although advertising is critical to attract new clients, mature organizations should also focus on getting existing clients to purchase more of the product themselves and to promote the product or service to their friends. Internal marketing is much less costly than mass media advertising and yields greater returns in sales volumes. Strategies to encourage referrals, for example, include rewarding loyal customers with free guest passes and discounts for bringing in new members.

Word of mouth is the most important way of attracting new members. Mullin, Hardy, and Sutton (1993) argue that if 70 percent of fitness sales come from word of mouth, and each satisfied consumer in turn refers .7 new customers, you may expect a total of 3.3 new referrals from a single word-of-mouth referral.

Advertising, however, is still necessary for a start-up organization or community program. Advertising is also necessary if you wish to attract new target groups, because word-of-mouth promotion by members will only reach people similar to themselves. The most common advertising strategies are mass media and mass mailings, both of which have a wide reach but are costly.

If you use mass media strategies, such as radio, television, or newspaper ads, consider the extent to which your intended audience is likely to be exposed to each medium. For instance, young adults are more likely to listen to late evening rock stations, and older adults are more likely to listen to daytime radio programming. Exposure alone, however, is no guarantee that the audience will pay attention to your message. According to a consumer survey, Brooks (1994) found people want advertising that portrays real people and realistic results.

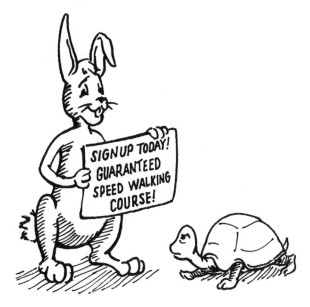

Captive audiences are much easier to reach than the general public, and promotional materials can be more personalized. Examples of captive audiences are work sites, schools, residential complexes, and senior's centers. Public health wellness programs are often taken directly to captive audiences, or, they may recruit from these existing groups. For instance, CHAMPS (Community Health Activities Model Program for Seniors) targeted a senior's center and a housing complex to promote activity options available in the community (Sepsis et al. 1995). A variety of promotional strategies were used, including posted flyers on bulletin boards, newsletter articles, presentations, and personalized invitations. These strategies were followed by introductory meetings, bringing in motivational peer speakers, and one-on-one assistance to help seniors select and register in community exercise programs of their choice. Evaluation showed that, for this audience, the introductory meetings and personal attention from project staff were perceived as highly motivating; T-shirts and prizes were not (Sepsis et al. 1995).

As noted in earlier in the chapter, you can segment potential consumers by several criteria in addition to demographic characteristics. Psychography—attitudes and lifestyles—may be one of the most important characteristics from a marketing perspective. Finding out where people in your area spend their time, such as malls or social clubs, can assist in personalizing recruitment efforts.

Regardless of whether you use mass advertising or go after more captive audiences, however, you must tailor promotional messages to people's attitudes and practices. Grantham et al. (1998) estimate that only about 15 percent of the population are hard core fitness enthusiasts. About 20 percent, meanwhile, are nonbelievers. Health promoters refer to this group as precontemplators. Regardless of the label, these individuals don't feel exercise is important for them and are simply not interested or ready to change their lifestyles. Health promoters have learned that activity promotion efforts targeting this segment are largely unsuccessful.

The majority of people, however, hold positive attitudes toward exercise, believe that exercise is important, and would like to be more active. This large segment, about two-thirds of the population, is being aggressively pursued by both the public health and the commercial sectors. This segment has been described as contemplators, uninitiated believers, and fence sitters. Tailoring promotional messages specifically to this segment has shown promising results.

*T*he Imagine Action campaign was promoted through work sites, schools, organizations, and media channels (Marcus et al. 1992). Based on whether people said they were thinking about being more active, exercising sporadically, or finding it hard to stick to a regular routine, they were sent specific materials. The first group was sent a booklet "What's In It For You" focusing on the benefits of active lifestyles and rewarding oneself. The second group was sent "Ready for Action" on how to set goals and time management. The third group was sent "Keep It Going" focusing on cross-training, avoiding injury, and trouble shooting. The campaign was successful in increasing and maintaining the activity level of people reached by the promotion.

Whatever promotional strategies you use, determine whether your strategies are cost-effective. How many people were exposed to the promotion, how many calls did you get as a result, how many joined your program or facility? It is much easier to evaluate extent of exposure or market penetration when targeting captive audiences, such as work sites, versus the general public. At a minimum, you should ask new members how they heard about the program. You can obtain a demographic and lifestyle profile of joiners through a simple background questionnaire. You can also survey visitors or guests who come into your facility but choose not to join, to obtain a profile of these exposed nonenrollers.

Perceptions of Facility and Program Features

Once people walk through your door as visitors or guests, they become potential consumers. Brooks (1994) found that features of fitness clubs that people found appealing included low-pressure sales tactics, trial memberships, reasonable prices, friendly and helpful staff and members, cleanliness, user-friendly equipment, and classes geared to their age and skill level. Being conscious of facility and program factors that may intimidate prospective members is important.

In Brooks' consumer survey, four sources of intimidation discouraged people from joining fitness clubs. They are

1. physical sources, such as fear of injury or lack of skill;

2. intellectual sources, such as difficulty operating fitness equipment;

3. psychological and social sources, such as feeling like outsiders; and

4. ethical sources, such as high-pressure sales tactics.

Many other examples would fit under each category. For instance, people may feel intimidated by the workout attire and physiques of staff and members. In fact, self-consciousness or feeling uncomfortable is one of the top barriers to activity in population surveys (CFLRI 1996d).

Similarity to existing members and to instructors in terms of age, gender, ethnicity, and abilities may be a consideration for some people. In particular, young instructors may intimidate some middle-aged and older clients. Special instruction or certification for working with older adults is recommended (Cotton, Ekeroth, and Yancy 1998; Grantham et al. 1998).

The extent to which screening procedures such as exercise stress testing, questionnaires such as the PARQ (Physical Activity Readiness Questionnaire), and medical clearance constitute barriers to participation is unknown, but it is a possibility all programs should consider.

Consumers may have a difficult time reconciling public health messages that exercise is safe and beneficial with the requirements of physician approval before they are allowed to participate. This may be especially true for older adults who tend to perceive exercise as risky (O'Brien Cousins and Vertinsky 1991). Also, not all physicians are convinced that exercise is safe for their patients, particularly those who are elderly and have chronic health problems (Myers 1987; Wilson et al. 1992). In any case, the more steps you ask people to take—fill out forms, book a checkup, see their doctor, and return the form—the less likely they are to comply.

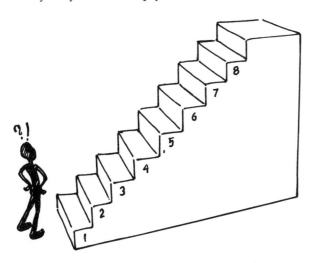

Many other facility and program features present potential barriers to exercise participation—noise level and overcrowding to name a few. Worksheet 2.1 provides an extensive checklist for programs to consider possible barriers inherent in their facilities and programs.

Consumer Attitudes and Expectations

As noted earlier, surveys indicate that most people hold positive attitudes toward exercise.

However, good intentions do not always translate into desirable behavior. Individuals who come to exercise programs and facilities are already motivated—they have taken the first step. Focusing on consumer expectations as opposed to general attitudes toward exercise is more useful for fitness marketing.

Analysis of four household surveys conducted in the United States and Canada (Stephens 1988) found that the number one reason cited for being physically active during leisure time was to feel better mentally and physically. The second and third most frequently cited reasons for being active were to control weight or look better and to relax or reduce stress. Similarly, Brooks (1994) found that the primary reasons cited for joining a fitness club were improving appearance (particularly losing weight and toning up), improving health, and feeling good.

For young women, concerns about weight, body image, and appearance are important (Myers, Weigel, and Holliday 1989). We are now finding that many aging women share similar concerns (O'Brien Cousins and Horne 1998). Younger men may want to build muscle mass; aging men may be concerned that their strength and athletic prowess are decreasing (O'Brien Cousins and Horne 1998). Once people reach middle age, preventing health problems, such as heart disease for men and osteoporosis for women, becomes more important (Myers, Weigel, and Holliday 1989).

Harada (1994) found that seniors in Japan said they were active for better health, relaxation, and meeting people. Similarly, we found that older adults in Canada gave a variety of reasons for joining exercise programs, including encouragement by friends (who were participating), to get out of the house, for fun and enjoyment, to meet people, and to keep healthy and active (Myers et al. in press). Health-related reasons were sometimes general, such as to delay the aging process, and sometimes specific, such as for my joints, for my arthritis, to sleep better, have more energy.

As people age, somatic complaints (sleeping disturbances, low energy levels, stiffness, and constipation) become more common. A significant proportion of middle-aged adults report sleep and other physical complaints. Health conditions and a sedentary lifestyle exacerbate these symptoms. Over time, exercise participation may lead to noticeable changes for people who have

Worksheet 2.1
Checklist of Potential Barriers

Accessibility

Is parking available? ☐ no ☐ yes On site ☐ or nearby ☐ ? Free ☐ or charge ☐ ?

Is site on a public transportation route? ☐ no ☐ yes   Stop nearby? ☐ no ☐ yes

Is site serviced by special (disabled) transport service(s)? ☐ no ☐ yes

Is site accessible by bicycle? ☐ no ☐ yes   Bike racks available? ☐ no ☐ yes

How is walking terrain in the area? ☐ good (even ground, sidewalks) ☐ poor

Are there stairs up to the entrance or exercise room? ☐ no ☐ yes (# flights ____ handrails ____)

Is entrance wheelchair or walker accessible (ramps)? ☐ no ☐ yes

Are parking areas, walkways, bike racks, and entrances well lit at night? ☐ no ☐ yes

Are entrances and walkways level or even? ☐ no ☐ yes

Is snow or ice removed from entrance areas when applicable? ☐ no ☐ yes

Is the area considered safe for walking alone? ☐ no ☐ yes ☐ unsure

Do you charge an initiation fee? ☐ no ☐ yes   Annual dues? ☐ no ☐ yes

Are there separate program or class fees? ☐ no ☐ yes   Pay as you go system? ☐ no ☐ yes

Are facility or class payment options or plans available? ☐ no ☐ yes

Do clients need to purchase equipment (e.g., squash goggles)? ☐ no ☐ yes

Is equipment available through loan? ☐ no ☐ yes   Or rental? ☐ no ☐ yes

Is specific clothing or footware needed? ☐ no ☐ yes

Are there screening procedures for new clients? ☐ no ☐ yes

Do you routinely give a medical form to new participants? ☐ no ☐ yes

Is signed physician permission or approval required? ☐ no ☐ yes

Do new clients sign a liability waiver? ☐ no ☐ yes

Facility Features

Is there an information desk? ☐ no ☐ yes

Are personnel assigned to welcome new members? ☐ no ☐ yes

Are personnel assigned to orient new members to the facility or equipment? ☐ no ☐ yes

Are fitness appraisals available? ☐ no ☐ yes   At an additional charge? ☐ no ☐ yes

Are change rooms or locker rooms available? ☐ no ☐ yes   With showers? ☐ no ☐ yes

Do the change rooms or locker rooms get crowded? ☐ no ☐ yes

Are towels provided? ☐ no ☐ yes

Are change rooms and exercise areas kept clean? ☐ no ☐ yes

Exercise Area

Is it easy to find the exercise area or pool? ☐ no ☐ yes

Are washrooms nearby? ☐ no ☐ yes   Sufficient number? ☐ no ☐ yes

Is a drinking fountain or cooler nearby? ☐ no ☐ yes

Is the exercise area well lit? ☐ no ☐ yes   Too dim ☐ or too much glare? ☐

Is the area well ventilated? ☐ no ☐ yes   Temperature control system? ☐ no ☐ yes

Are there competing activities in the area? ☐ no ☐ yes   Competing noise? ☐ no ☐ yes

Is overcrowding an issue for classes, the weight room, the pool, etc.? ☐ no ☐ yes

If you have a pool, is temperature closely monitored? ☐ no ☐ yes

If you have a pool, is it accessible by stairway with handrails? ☐ no ☐ yes

Class Features

Do participants have a choice of class days or times? ☐ no ☐ yes

Ratio of participants to instructor(s) and assistants? _____ to _____

Gender of instructor(s)? ☐ male ☐ female ☐ both

Gender ratio of participants? _____ number of males to _____ number of females

Age of instructor(s) _____   Age range of participants _____ to _____

Do you give participants options for exercise intensity or self-pacing? ☐ no ☐ yes

Do you teach participants to monitor their heart rates? ☐ no ☐ yes

Can all participants easily observe the instructor? ☐ no ☐ yes

Can all participants easily hear the instructor? ☐ no ☐ yes

Do you use music in the class? ☐ no ☐ yes

Have you consulted participants regarding type and volume of music? ☐ no ☐ yes

Is there a gathering area (outside exercise room with seating)? ☐ no ☐ yes

Are there opportunities for socializing? ☐ before ☐ during ☐ after class

previously been inactive (Myers et al. in press). For regularly active individuals, such symptoms may only become noticeable if their exercise routine is disrupted (Schneider 1996).

Program deliverers should heed the consistent findings concerning the primary expectations of most fitness consumers—to look and feel better. We will return to these findings in chapter 5 when discussing selection of client-outcome measures.

Before we leave the section on exercise adoption, it is important to mention that habitual exercisers, especially elite athletes, are more informed consumers and have different expectations when choosing fitness facilities. Such individuals are unlikely to be intimidated by fitness equipment or vigorous training. In fact, for them, sophisticated exercise equipment may be an important feature in choosing one training facility over another. Coaching and available competition may be other important considerations in selecting a sports club. Concerning older athletes, O'Brien Cousins and Burgess (1992) caution that

Table 2.1 Factors Influencing Exercise Adoption and Adherence

Client factors	Environmental factors	Program and facility factors
Demographics (age, gender, and education)	Community options (availability and accessibility)	Advertisment
		Accessibility
Resources (discretionary income and transportation)	Social support (family, friends, and physicians)	Costs and payment plans
Other responsibilities and time management	Weather and safety concerns	Orientations, services, and amenities
Lifestyle and health (exercise behavior, smoking, weight, mobility limitations)		Appearance, cleanliness, and comfort
		Screening procedures
Cognition (readiness, attitudes, awareness, outcome expectations, self-efficacy expectations)		Activity options, scheduling, and pacing
		Characteristics of exercise leaders and coparticipants
		Opportunities to socialize

coaches need to be aware of and sensitive to different expectations for sport performance (i.e., maintenance rather than progress), as well as opportunities to have fun and socialize.

Finally, a few words on constraints to initiating physical activity. Not surprisingly, frequently reported barriers to physical activity that people cite are time or competing priorities; cost and transportation; lack of energy, motivation, interest; lack of exposure and skills; feeling uncomfortable or self-conscious; illness or injury; and fear of injury or exercising in unsafe places (Brooks 1994; CFLRI 1996d). Less active individuals may require the encouragement of a friend, partner, or physician (Brooks 1994). Older women, in particular, report lack of an exercise companion as a barrier to participation (O'Brien Cousins 1998).

Social support has been identified as an important factor influencing exercise adoption and adherence (Clark 1996; Courneya and McAuley 1995; O'Brien Cousins 1998). Social influences, however, can be positive or negative (facilitating or inhibiting). Family members, friends, and physicians can either encourage or discourage initiating and maintaining physical activity. Some individuals join fitness clubs or community programs because of their friends or partners, others to meet new people, still others because of the camaraderie or fellowship that develops in a class or group setting (Carron, Widmeyer, and Brawley 1988; Schneider 1996; Spink and Carron 1992). Exercise instructors can provide direct support and opportunities to socialize and build group cohesion to foster exercise adherence.

Table 2.1 summarizes the many personal, environmental, and program factors that can influence exercise participation. Some factors, as discussed in the previous section, are instrumental in exercise initiation. Other factors, discussed in the next section, are important for adherence. Several factors, such as social support, influence both adoption and adherence.

Factors Influencing Program Adherence

Once people join a fitness facility or community exercise program or enlist the services of a personal trainer, the challenge is to keep them. This section summarizes what we have learned about exercise adherence through research and tracking participants of programs and fitness clubs.

First, we define adherence. Then, we examine predictors of adherence and motivational techniques leaders can use to retain participants.

Defining Adherence

Dishman (1994) broadly defines *adherence* as "the level of participation achieved in a behavioral regimen once the individual has agreed to undertake it" (p. 186). The word adherence means to stick to something. It is often used to describe a person's continuation in an exercise program. The terms adherence and retention are interchangeable. Likewise, nonadherence, attrition, and dropout—all referring to losing clients—are interchangeable.

It is much easier to verbally describe adherence than to operationally define and measure it. The next chapter provides formulas to calculate attendance and dropout rates. Now let's look at adherence rates that have been reported in the exercise field. You can use these rates as *benchmarks,* or a basis of comparison, to see how well you are doing relative to similar programs with similar clientele.

Benchmarks of Adherence

For health and fitness clubs, the annual, average attrition rate (or loss of members) is somewhere between 34 percent and 38 percent (Grantham et al. 1998; Mullin, Hardy, and Sutton 1993); however, it is not uncommon for clubs to exceed 50 percent. A club with a 50 percent attrition rate would need to bring in new sales of 60 percent to achieve a 10 percent growth in membership.

Although each club must determine its own member attrition rates (see chapter 3), Grantham et al. (1998) suggest that fitness clubs compare themselves to the national industry standard of about 35 percent. They suggest that less than 10 percent annual attrition is excellent, and 11 percent to 21 percent is good.

As noted in chapter 1, we know more about adherence of younger adults to aerobic training programs than about other groups or types of programs. Adherence by young adults to structured, high-intensity aerobic classes is generally poor. About 50 percent of joiners drop out in the first three to six months, most in the first 12 weeks (Dishman and Sallis 1994). Many exercise studies and programs compare their dropout rates to this well-known benchmark.

There is some evidence that adherence may be better for moderate- than high-intensity aerobic exercise and for home-based than class-based regimens (King et al. 1991). Obvious advantages of home-based exercise include convenience; flexibility of scheduling; and no costs for transportation, fees, or special attire (Dishman 1994; King et al. 1991).

In the cardiac rehabilitation area, Oldridge (1982) reports that the dropout rate for middle-aged males is approximately 30 percent in the first six months, but adherence increases over time—40 percent in their trials participated for a full four years. Extended tracking of middle-aged men shows good long-term adherence for motivated members of this clinical population (Oldridge 1982).

Persons with Type 2 or adult onset diabetes, who are likely to be overweight and have mobility problems, have much higher rates of exercise relapse (75 percent to 80 percent) compared with nondiabetics (Krug, Haire-Joshu, and Heady 1991). For our diabetes class, we found a decent average attendance rate (70 percent) while they were in the program, but the three-year dropout rate was high—about 75 percent (Ecclestone, Myers, and Patterson 1998).

It would be easy to conclude from the above findings that people with diabetes are poor exercise adherers. However, Schneider et al. (1992) conducted one-year follow-up interviews with 100 previously sedentary individuals with diabetes who had dropped out of a structured exercise program within the first three months. Almost three-quarters of these individuals reported that they were in fact exercising (on their own or in other classes) at least twice a week, suggesting that their brief structured commitment may have facilitated subsequent activity. We also found that some of our diabetes class dropouts joined other programs (Ecclestone, Myers, and Patterson 1998). This is an important finding that would have escaped the usual definition of adherence.

Thus, you should not label a participant an exercise dropout without follow-up to ascertain their activity behavior (Ecclestone, Myers, and Patterson 1998). Clinicians and public health specialists will be particularly pleased to hear this because their primary objective is to keep people active—no matter what activity they choose to do. Commercial clubs, meanwhile, are less interested that their members are continuing to exercise after they quit the club. However, they should be curious about why their members leave and if they go to their competitors. In chapter 6 I provide guidelines on how to contact and assess absent members or clients.

As I illustrate in chapter 3, establishing a database of attendance patterns for various classes can be useful. Using our database of 670 registrants in 12 different exercise programs at the Centre for Activity and Ageing, we tracked participation and dropout rates over a three-year period (Ecclestone, Myers, and Patterson 1998). Not unlike the results for younger groups, our data showed that most dropouts occur in the first 3 months; 75 percent of those who drop out do so by 6 months. However, after 12 months, only 8 percent more dropped out in the subsequent two years, illustrating the importance of extended tracking (Ecclestone, Myers, and Patterson 1998). Both attendance and adherence patterns varied considerably from class to class. For instance, although Tai Chi initially had a low enrollment, the class filled to capacity over a few months, average attendance was over 80 percent, and more than half of the original participants were still in the class three years later. We also found that people switched classes, and some who left for extended periods (for travel, health, caregiving, or other reasons), later rejoined their programs or recycled into other programs. Only long-term tracking can establish these patterns.

Predictors of Adherence

A number of demographic variables—higher education and income, male gender, younger age, healthy—have been associated with higher rates of physical activity (Dishman 1994). Conversely, obesity, smoking, chronic health problems, and advanced age are associated with being sedentary and act as disincentives for exercise adoption and adherence. Yet these are the people who may benefit most from exercise.

Both Minor and Brown (1993) and Rejeski et al. (1997) found that immediate past exercise behavior was the best predictor of future compliance. In other words, the longer people continue exercising, the more likely they will keep doing so. Neither study found that objective fitness results, such as increased aerobic capacity, predicted maintenance.

There is evidence that if people see quick results, they are more likely to continue exercising.

This has been demonstrated concerning weight loss in individuals with diabetes (cf. Raz, Hauser, and Bursztyn 1994), perceived pain reduction in those with arthritis (cf. Minor and Brown 1993), and noticeable improvements in sleep and energy levels in the general public (Myers et al. in press).

When the initial experience is over, and persons undertake their own exercise routine, habit becomes key (Minor and Brown 1993). People learn to overcome obstacles, such as bad weather or not feeling well, and develop strategies to maintain their exercise routines—provided they feel they are benefiting from exercise.

Motivational Considerations

Outcome expectations—what people hope to get from exercise—appear to be important for exercise initiation (Rodgers and Brawley 1991). For instance, those with diabetes may need to believe that exercise will lead to weight loss and better glycemic control. People with arthritis may need to believe that exercise will relieve and not aggravate joint pain, or young people may need to believe that exercise can take inches off their hips or waist. In any case, outcome expectations must be realistic and attainable in the short term.

Self-efficacy expectations also affect exercise adoption and adherence (Dishman 1994). Self-efficacy expectations refer to one's self-confidence in specific areas (Bandura 1977, 1997). For instance, a person may be confident she can keep up with an aquafit class but not with a high-intensity aerobic class. Someone else may be confident he can ride a bike but not that he can swim the length of a pool. People tend to avoid situations for which they distrust their skills or capabilities. Self-efficacy plays an important role until the exercise behavior becomes routine or habitual and when one's routine is disrupted (McAuley, Lox, and Duncan 1993). Measures of self-efficacy are reviewed in chapter 5.

Through progressive and realistic goal setting and by providing positive feedback concerning accomplishments, exercise leaders can play an important role in enhancing participants' self-efficacy. Helping participants correctly interpret exercise sensations, such as sweating, rapid breathing, and muscle soreness, is also important. For instance, a cardiac patient not used to exercising may interpret normal sensations as signs of angina (Ewart et al. 1986).

Leadership style and program pacing can enhance or reduce participants' self-confidence. For instance, anxiety may be "reinforced by the leader who gives patronage to old notions about overexerting the body and diligently conducts heart-rate monitoring every few minutes" (O'Brien Cousins and Burgess 1992, 465). Participants who feel pressured to keep up may quickly become frustrated or injured.

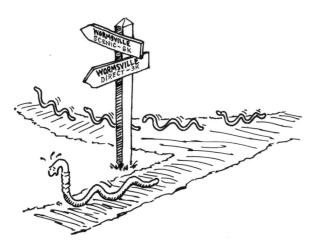

O'Brien Cousins and Burgess (1992) discuss the importance of exercise leaders constantly being observant of their participants. For instance, exercise leaders should listen for a buzz after an announcement as an indication that participants didn't clearly hear the instructions and are asking others around them what they are supposed to do. Diligent observation is critical to ensure that clients follow self-pacing, especially when classes consist of individuals with mixed abilities. Instructors can also underestimate the capabilities of their participants. As one participant quipped to her instructor, "We were wondering how long it would take you to figure out most of us could handle much more" (p. 471).

Past experiences with exercise influence outcome and efficacy expectations. Recollections of childhood experiences can build or undermine self-efficacy in adulthood. Interested readers are referred to O'Brien Cousins (1998). Exercise leaders working with older adults need to be aware that the current generation of older men may have a history of militaristic calisthenics and competitive male-only team sports in their youth (Harada 1994; Tudor-Locke and Myers 1998). In contrast, many women from this generation are trying new physical activities for the first time. Their history likely includes little sports skill training (O'Brien Cousins and Vertinsky 1991); displays of athleticism were considered unfeminine and tomboyish. Before the 1920s, the social convention that women cover their bodies precluded swimwear conducive to swimming. Many older women depend on their husbands as leisure instigators and partners; widows may be reluctant to go out and exercise alone (O'Brien Cousins 1998).

Exercise leaders need to be sensitive to generational attitudes and experiences. At the same time, however, leaders should not assume that people will not try new things. For instance, one might not expect that older adults, especially older women, would be interested in weight training, yet the weight rooms at our Centre for Activity and Ageing are filled with both men and women. The key is to get people to try several exercise options till they find the ones that are right for them. We found that people who tried several different exercise classes versus just one class were more likely to stay at the Centre over the long term (Ecclestone, Myers, and Patterson 1998).

Motivational techniques are critical to foster exercise adherence. For instance, Minor and Brown (1993) incorporated personal feedback, goal setting, and opportunity to include partners—strategies similar to those employed by many exercise programs. Rejeski et al. (1997) went even further—subjects were offered transportation to and from the clinic, home visits, telephone contact, and, for resistance training at home, the opportunity to exchange weights as they became stronger. The feasibility of such intensive motivational techniques, however, is doubtful for nonresearch programs.

Even brief telephone contact of staff with absent members may promote adherence (Hillsdon and Thorogood 1996; Wankel and Thompson 1977). Fostering group cohesion in class-based programs and encouraging buddy systems are also practical social support strategies instructors can use to enhance adherence (Spink and Carron 1992).

Some people may enjoy exercising with people of different ages; others may prefer exercise companions of similar age. Still others prefer unstructured, solitary exercise. Similarly, people differ in their preferences for gender-integrated versus gender-segregated exercise classes. Many of our classes have both men and women. The Men's Retirement Association is an example of a successful age- and gender-segregated group. This group currently has 100 members and an annual attrition rate of less than 8 percent. What's interesting is when some of their wives wanted to join, they were told to form their own association. Today, the women's retirement exercise class has 80 members who exercise at the same time as the men, but at opposite ends of the track!

Fun, enjoyment of the activity, and camaraderie with group members are themes that emerge repeatedly in focus groups with older men and women. Filling the void created by retirement and feelings of accomplishment were additional reasons for adherence in a men's retirement group (Tudor-Locke and Myers 1998). Similar personal testimonials from older exercisers appear in Van Norman Van Norman (1995):

> **O**ne gentleman who had been in the same water aerobics class for nine years was asked why he prefers this class. He responded, "Music I enjoy listening to and an instructor that has enthusiasm for teaching are important to me. Our group of early birds . . . It's a great way to start the day with people you have come to know and enjoy. If I miss a week or two, I notice a definite pain and stiffness in my muscles and joints" (p. 4).

Working clients may be too busy to socialize before or after exercise classes, as may some retired adults. For instance, we found that participants in rural areas used after-class time as an opportunity to socialize, but urban class participants wanted to get in and out as quickly as possible. Determine the extent to which opportunities to socialize and areas to congregate before and after class are important to your clientele.

Obviously, some factors that influence exercise adoption and adherence are more under the control of exercise leaders than others. According to surveys of commercial fitness facilities, approximately 70 percent of the reasons people leave these facilities are controllable (Grantham et al. 1998). Examples include poor facility or equipment management, appearance, programming, scheduling, crowding, and instructor encouragement. Conversely, uncontrollable factors include job or financial changes, extended illness, and family interruptions such as birth or moving out of the area (Grantham et al. 1998). Other factors, such as opportunities for socialization, age- and gender-integrated versus segregated programming, music selection, and pacing, are also things that exercise leaders can modify. Evaluation can help you identify which factors are important to your clientele so you can tailor programs to better meet their needs and expectations.

Summary

It is important to be aware of patterns and projections in the exercise field. However, you need to collect your own information to determine how your clients compare with consumer profiles in similar sectors and whether your client profile changes over time. Social marketing techniques, particularly segmentation, are useful if you wish to expand your client base. Before jumping on the bandwagon and purchasing the latest equipment or starting new programs, however, you first need to conduct an evaluation to determine the size of your potential market, the number and nature of existing services, and the level of interest among your target audience. I describe needs assessment or market analysis in chapter 4.

All exercise leaders want to attract and keep clients. Understanding factors that may influence exercise adoption and adherence is important. However, you still need to identify barriers inherent in your programs and expectations and preferences of your clientele. Adherence rates found by others can serve as a basis of comparison, but only if you track your own rates of adherence. Chapter 3 shows you how.

Working Exercises

1. Use the checklist in worksheet 2.1 to consider which factors may potentially inhibit people from joining your program and which factors may contribute to dropout. Highlight the factors you are able to do something about or change.

2. Write a description of your intended target audiences (i.e., who you would like to reach).

3. Then, write a description of your clientele (i.e., who is coming to your program).

4. List the motivational techniques you presently use to enhance participation rates and adherence. Do you have a standard procedure for contacting absent members?

5. Think about how you define or describe a dropout in your program.

6. Do you currently record dropout rates? If so, describe how. Chapter 3 provides assistance.

Customizing Your Client-Information Systems

Chapter 1 explored what you and other stake-holders would like to know about your program and participants. After reading chapter 2, you may be curious about how your membership growth, client profile, and adherence rates compare with similar sectors of the fitness industry. Evaluation is necessary to determine how well your program is doing in attracting, retaining, and meeting the expectations of your clientele. Evaluation helps you make strategic choices in collecting information based on what you want to know and what is most useful for decision making. Programs need to develop their own customized information system.

This chapter examines the status quo or typical record-keeping practices of exercise programs. Most fitness programs do head counts, but do not systematically track patterns of growth and adherence or monitor usage patterns (Grantham et al. 1998). Typically, enrollment and participation rates are aggregated across a class or several classes. Programs often do not know how dropouts differ from adherers and which types of clients improve the most. Also, client-satisfaction surveys are the norm for soliciting participant feedback.

Many fitness organizations "have only a *superficial* idea of the demographic breakdown of their memberships and crude *guesstimates* of total head counts" (Mullin, Hardy, and Sutton 1993, 93, italics added).

As you read this chapter, compare your record-keeping practices with the status quo. Think about the types of information you would like to have, but do not currently collect. Think about all the information you do collect but never use for decision making. Consider how your clients would react if they knew how little the program uses the information they supply through registration forms, medical histories, fitness appraisals, and satisfaction questionnaires. How many times have you asked yourself, "Does anyone ever look at this or do they just pitch it?" How many quarterly or annual reports sit on your shelves gathering dust?

Most programs have record-keeping procedures for payrolls, equipment purchases, and client payments. As programs increase in size, they

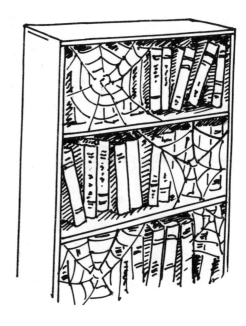

are more likely to use simple computer spreadsheets for recording and tabulating financial data. Programs may also electronically file and update client mailing lists. Even large programs, however, often store most client information (such as liability waivers, medical histories, and fitness appraisals) manually, in separate folders for each person. Attendance sheets tend to be filed by program and aggregated across participants. Client-satisfaction questionnaires, meanwhile, are usually filed in batches according to when they were compiled (e.g., 1999 surveys, 2000 surveys).

Collecting information at one point in time can provide a snapshot picture of your client profile, usage rates, or satisfaction ratings. To examine patterns or trends, however, you must take several snapshots. Recording and comparing information over time is referred to as _monitoring_ or _tracking_. To compare different sources of information, such as which clients participate more often, which clients show the most improvement, or which clients tend to drop out, you need a system that allows you to link separate sources of information.

> **A** customized system tailored for your program puts client information at your fingertips to compare, link, and track patterns over time.

This book shows you step-by-step how to develop a client-information system customized to meet your evaluation needs, using the resources at your disposal. The first step is sorting through your current information-gathering practices to determine whether they are adequate or need to be modified to yield more useful and accessible information.

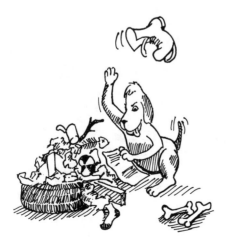

Head Counts

Most programs or facilities can tell you how many participants or members they have at a given time (usually over the past year). As Mullin, Hardy, and Sutton (1993) note, however, these head counts may be only guesstimates.

For clubs or fitness facilities, payment of initiation fees is the easiest way to determine the number of new members. Payment of annual dues or renewal forms is the easiest way to determine the number of continuing members, and conversely, the number who discontinue their membership. For other types of programs or services, you can use payment of session, class, or service fees to determine numbers of new and continuing clients. Exercise programs and facilities that are not fee based may rely on registrations and logs, such as sign-in sheets, to determine the number of new and continuing clients, respectively.

At a minimum, Grantham et al. (1998) recommend that fitness facilities and clubs keep track of

1. membership growth (MG),
2. member attrition rate (percent) (MA), and
3. average length of membership (ALM).

Grantham and colleagues suggest the following formulas:

$$MG = \text{number of new members who join over a given period} - \text{number of terminations over the same period}$$

$$MA = (\text{number of members lost during period} \div \text{number of members at start of period}) \times 100$$

$$ALM = \frac{1}{MA}$$

Using the first formula, the net difference represents either a positive or negative growth rate. Grantham et al. (1998) recommend that all fitness clubs tabulate member growth and attrition monthly and annually to examine fluctuations. By comparing the data over time, referred to as _tracking_, facilities can begin to see patterns and trends. You can use this information to plan sales promotions during periods of low volume and adjust staffing accordingly, or to plan special events for certain times of the year.

You can also compare your rates of membership growth, attrition, and duration to market survey findings. For instance, the industry standard of 35 percent attrition (described in chapter 2) yields an average length of membership of 2.85 years. If a club improves their attrition rate to 20 percent, using the third formula shows that the average length of membership increases to 5.00 years (Grantham et al. 1998).

Although useful, these formulas represent an overly simplistic picture. For instance, how do you determine when a member is considered lost? Short of resignation letters, it is not always easy to determine if a client has left your club, program, or service for good. Members who do not renew or pay annual dues on time are not usually terminated outright, but are sent reminder letters and may be assessed late penalties. Each facility needs to establish criteria for termination or closure. For example, members will be considered to have terminated membership if payment is not received within one month following the second reminder letter sent by registered mail. A clear and consistent policy has several advantages. First, such criteria help you calculate accurate attrition rates. Second, members are less likely to complain about inequitable standards because the same policy applies to everyone.

In session-based programs, clients may not renew for the next session, but may return for subsequent sessions. In ongoing programs, some participants leave for extended periods, but later return to the program. Because we have multiple, ongoing programs, we decided to define a *dropout* as a person "not being registered in any of the Centre programs, not attending a single session over a 12-month period, and not returning to any class at the Centre for a subsequent 12-month period" (Ecclestone, Myers, and Patterson 1998, 75).

As noted in chapter 2, dropout is not a term that is simple to *operationalize*, or to define and measure. Different programs use different definitions. For instance, according to Oldridge (1982), "dropout implies that an individual is no longer participating in the program at the specified minimal frequency" (p. 56). In their heart health program, a person was considered a dropout if he had not attended a single supervised session for eight weeks for reasons other than cardiac events or death (Oldridge 1979).

According to the definitions used by Oldridge and my colleagues, it is necessary to keep track of individual attendance patterns to calculate dropout rates across clients. The next section illustrates the advantages of individual attendance recording as opposed to aggregate records.

Aggregate User Rates

Although initial enrollment may be high, this indicator is no guarantee that people continue coming to a program. User rates are important to profit and nonprofit programs alike. Low enrollment and low participation rates often determine whether a class will continue. Conversely, high participation rates and other indicators of demand, such as waiting lists, justify additional classes, and high usage rates justify equipment purchases.

Grantham et al. (1998) recommend that all fitness facilities closely monitor user rates and high versus low usage periods (days of the week, times of the day). User rates are easier to record for group-based classes (attendance taking), but you can record them for almost anything, for instance, using manual sign-up sheets for treadmill users or logs for pool use. Technology—computerized check-in systems, bar code scanners, and the fingerprint and voice recognition methods promised in the new millennium—can assist in the tracking process.

Exercise programs are more likely to record average attendance or aggregate user rates (AUR) than individual attendance rates. The following formula is easy to use:

AUR = (the total number of users ÷ the total

number of sessions or opportunities)

× 100

The top of table 3.1 shows a simple example of average attendance based on head counts for five classes. In this example, the average or aggregate attendance rate is 72 percent.

Aggregate user rates can tell you about overall usage patterns, such as whether attendance is higher on Mondays than Fridays, whether attendance rates are consistent over time, and how usage compares for different classes or services.

Table 3.1 Aggregate Versus Individual Attendance Recording

	Class 1	Class 2	Class 3	Class 4	Class 5
Aggregate attendance	10	8	6	8	4
Average = 7.2/class					

Individual attendance recording						
	Class 1	Class 2	Class 3	Class 4	Class 5	Indiv. rate
1. Mrs. Jones	✓	✓	✓	✓	✓	100%
2. Mr. Smith	✓	✓	–	–	–	40%
3. Mr. Brown	✓	–	–	–	–	20%
4. Mrs. Black	✓	✓	✓	✓	–	80%
5. Mrs. White	✓	–	✓	✓	✓	80%
6. Mrs. Reynolds	✓	✓	–	✓	✓	80%
7. Ms. Patrick	✓	✓	–	✓	–	60%
8. Mrs. Maki	✓	✓	✓	✓	–	80%
9. Mrs. Ross	✓	✓	✓	✓	–	80%
10. Mrs. Reid	✓	✓	✓	✓	✓	100%
Total	10	8	6	8	4	
Average = 72%						

However, aggregate rates based on total head counts do not tell you anything about the users themselves.

There is a great deal more that you can learn about your program and your clientele by recording *individual* participation or usage rates as opposed to relying on total head counts.

Individual participation rates allow you to determine which classes or equipment are most popular for male versus female clients, working versus retired clients, and so on. You can also detect patterns of absence and identify clients who may be getting ready to leave and need a motivational boost such as a phone call (Mullin, Hardy, and Sutton 1993). You can more accurately calculate dropout. You can compare characteristics of continued users with characteristics of dropouts. Equally important, you can examine the extent of client improvement or outcomes according to participation rates.

Table 3.1 compares the information that you can obtain from individual versus aggregate attendance recording. As you can see, the total numbers or head counts for each class are identical, as is the average attendance rate. By visually examining the individual attendance pattern, you can see that only 2 of the 10 participants attended all five sessions. Participant 3 stopped coming after the first class, and participant 2 stopped coming after the second class. Interestingly, both are men in an otherwise all-female class. As this is a small data set, you would not want to draw too many conclusions. However, it does illustrate possible patterns that you would not detect through more limited aggregate attendance recording. Chapter 7 shows you how to track participation and adherence patterns using a larger data set.

In the right-hand column of table 3.1, you will notice that an individual attendance rate (IAR) has been calculated for each of the 10 participants in this class.

IAR = (number of sessions attended by the person ÷ total number of sessions offered) × 100

Is it important to note that you easily determine the average participation rate from individual attendance records. The reverse, however, is not true. If you do only head counts (as shown in the top of table 3.1), you have no way of knowing whether the same people came to different classes. Individual attendance information is also necessary to accurately determine dropout rates. Each program, however, will need to decide how they wish to use this information. For instance, because our clients pay monthly fees (classes run three times a week), we chose to examine participation rates on a class by class as well as a monthly basis (Ecclestone, Myers, and Patterson 1998). Recall that in our formula to calculate dropout rate, we did not include clients who did not attend a single session over the month under examination. As in the above formula, we were careful not to include cancelled sessions in the denominator in order not to underestimate the rate of participation. If your program has a different scenario (for example, a 12-week prenatal exercise class, or a 6-week

weight-training group), consider examining participation and dropout rates over 12-week and 6-week periods, respectively, rather than over a monthly period. Chapter 6 discusses practical strategies for tracking participation rates for large fitness facilities with multiple classes and services.

Ultimately, you need to decide what constitutes acceptable participation and retention rates for your programs. You can compare your rates with those of other facilities serving the same market, as well as across your programs and over time within a program, to monitor trends.

Client Profiles

Although each instructor may know a great deal about the individuals in his or her class or service, most organizations have only a vague idea of the demographic breakdown of their memberships. A more detailed profile of your clientele is necessary to achieve the following:

- Determine who you are attracting to your programs.
- Compare high- and low-frequency users.
- Compare characteristics of adherers and dropouts.
- Examine which types of clients improve the most.
- Compare whether your client profile changes over time.
- Compare your clientele to similar sectors of the industry.

When clients first join, they typically fill out a registration form and a medical history. Many facilities offer fitness appraisals and individual goal setting as member services for screening and motivational purposes. You can also use this information to develop client profiles and to examine extent of change across your clientele and over time.

When the Centre for Activity and Ageing began a three-year tracking study of registrants, gender and age were the only characteristics routinely recorded for all participants. We found interesting patterns of both attendance and adherence based on age and gender, but wished we had more information about our clientele.

We now routinely administer a more detailed background questionnaire to each new registrant. The forms we use to collect client information are customized for our Centre programs and for each of our outreach programs—community wellness clinics, Home Support Exercise Program, and Functional Fitness Long-Term Care Program. Chapter 6 contains a prototype of a background questionnaire to get you started and provides suggestions for customizing this form, depending on the nature of your programs and your clientele.

Client-Satisfaction Surveys

According to Grantham et al. (1998), "a previously commonplace tactic was to lure a prospect to become a member through payment in advance of an annual fee, then to discourage continued attendance through inattention and indifference" (p. 21). Consumers are more discriminating than ever before, and today's business practices focus on customer service. Studies show that it costs five times more to attract a new member than to retain an existing member (Grantham et al. 1998). Keeping clients satisfied is considered crucial for maintaining your revenue base and for obtaining word-of-mouth referrals.

Client-satisfaction surveys represent the status quo for obtaining participant feedback. In fact, such surveys frequently constitute the only formal evaluation many programs conduct. Such surveys are easy to design, and you can tailor them to examine the unique features of each program. Information is collected systematically in that everyone fills out the same form. Honest and objective reporting is enhanced because questionnaires are anonymous. Also, you can easily aggregate ratings for year-end reports or presentations to various stakeholders. Although

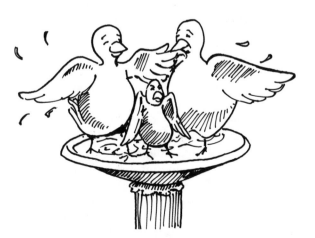

client-satisfaction surveys have many selling points, they also have several limitations, including response bias, representativeness, and interpretation.

Response Bias

Client-satisfaction ratings tend to be highly skewed toward the positive end of the rating scale. This tendency holds up whether the service in question is fast foods, health care, or exercise programming (Favaro 1995; Myers 1996). Some people may be hesitant to complain for fear of losing the service, or they do not want to ruin it for others, even if they personally haven't gotten much out of the program. Psychologists might explain this phenomenon as avoidance of cognitive dissonance (I'm still here, so I must be getting something out of it).

> **D**id you know that 80 percent to 85 percent of consumers will say they are moderately to highly satisfied, no matter what the service?

Another explanation that has received empirical support is that people consider the service deliverer (class instructor or personal trainer) more than any other feature of the program, and if they like the service deliverer, participants will generally give overall positive ratings to the program itself. Some trends that have emerged from consumer surveys of both profit and nonprofit services (Favaro 1995) are the following:

- About two-thirds of consumers say they switch services because of staff indifference.
- Satisfied consumers tell about three other people about their experience.
- Less than one-third of dissatisfied consumers make a formal complaint, but each is likely to tell 9 or 10 other people about the experience.

The first thing to note is that word-of-mouth comments about a program can either encourage or discourage personal referrals. Dissatisfied customers are more likely to tell their friends than the program itself about their bad experiences. Consumer studies also clearly show that people switch services of all kinds not because of the product or program, but because they feel hassled or ignored (Favaro 1995; Myers 1996). Being perceived as approachable, friendly, and well intentioned will earn instructors as many points and probably more points on a satisfaction rating scale than will their skills. In fact, it is debatable whether clients can judge the technical skills or competency of service providers, whether physicians, rehabilitation therapists, or exercise instructors, but they do know whether they receive caring and courteous treatment.

O'Brien Cousins and Burgess (1992) describe a long-established fitness class at a famous beach resort that attracts a loyal following year after year. The instructor and the participants were both from an older cohort, and the exercises themselves were right out of the World War II era: highly regimented, jerky, and hard on the joints—hardly what modern exercise specialists would recommend, especially for older adults. Nevertheless, these participants had a strong allegiance to this instructor and, had they been surveyed, would likely have given high satisfaction ratings.

A final reason that client-satisfaction results tend to be skewed is that participants who are dissatisfied, those for whom the program has not met their needs or expectations, are not around long enough to fill out your surveys!

Representativeness

Client-satisfaction questionnaires are typically distributed at the end of a program session (if the program is time limited) or at the end of the year (if the program is ongoing). In either case, only those present that day have the opportunity to complete the survey. Because such surveys tend to be anonymous, programs have no way of determining who filled them out.

Program dropouts are not represented in client-satisfaction surveys!

Less frequent participants also tend to be underrepresented in satisfaction surveys. Consider the following techniques for maximizing your response rate:

- Include an envelope for returning the survey to a drop-off box.
- Do not conduct your survey close to holiday periods.
- Designate more than one class for distributing the surveys.
- Have someone other than the class instructor distribute the surveys.
- Consider mailing the survey (with an addressed, postage paid envelope) to all registrants.

Programs should report the response rate when presenting client survey findings. For example, let's say that 100 people were registered in a Tai Chi program, but only 40 were there the day you handed out the survey. You get 20 back. Is your response rate 50 percent? It would be more accurate to use the total number registered in the class versus the number present the day of the survey to calculate response rate. Using the following formula, your response rate (RR) would be only 20 percent.

RR = (number returned ÷ total number of registrants) × 100

Interpretation

So, what do you do with the client-satisfaction surveys you get back? Most client-satisfaction questionnaires consist of two types of questions: forced-choice responses or open-ended comments. Forced-choice response rating formats often look like this,

0	1	2	3	4
Poor				Excellent

or like this:

1	2	3	4	5
Extremely dissatisfied	Moderately dissatisfied	Neither satisfied nor dissatisfied	Moderately satisfied	Extremely satisfied

A more creative rating format is illustrated in figure 3.1.

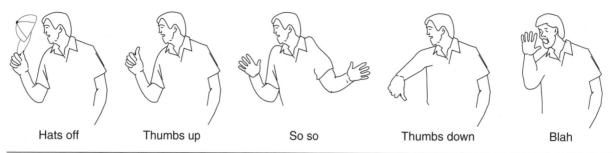

Hats off   Thumbs up   So so   Thumbs down   Blah

Figure 3.1 Satisfaction rating format.

Let's look at the results from a hypothetical client survey to illustrate how difficult it is to interpret such ratings, regardless of the rating format used. I've simplified the example in table 3.2 by using 100 respondents (to make calculating percentages easy). In this example, we will assume all respondents completed every question. Usually, at least some questionnaires contain missing data, in which case you need to divide the number of people who gave a particular rating by the total number of people (in each row) who answered the question; then multiply by 100. You can also combine or aggregate rating categories for presentation purposes. For instance, in this example, a total of 88 percent (28 + 60) said they were either moderately or extremely satisfied with the program instructor.

So, how might program personnel interpret and use the findings in table 3.2? Although there were mixed reactions to many elements of the program, programs might rationalize these findings on the grounds that you cannot please all the people all the time. They could take consolation in the finding that most participants (75 percent) were moderately to extremely satisfied with the program overall. In addition, almost three-quar-

Table 3.2 Possible Responses to a Client-Satisfaction Survey (100 Respondents)

How satisfied are you with the	1 Extremely dissatisfied	2 Moderately dissatisfied	3 Neither satisfied nor dissatisfied	4 Moderately satisfied	5 Extremely satisfied
program instructor?	0	0	12	28	60
exercises?	10	25	25	27	13
music?	0	12	18	45	25
location?	15	27	22	30	6
class schedule?	17	29	20	17	17
facility?	20	32	23	20	5
take home guide?	8	15	34	22	21
program overall?	0	10	15	45	30

Has this program met your expectations?	Yes = 72	No = 28
Do you feel you have benefited from this program?	Yes = 80	No = 20
Would you recommend this program to others?	Yes = 87	No = 13

ters felt that the program met their expectations, 80 percent felt that they had benefited from the program, and 87 percent said they would recommend the program to others.

Certainly, these findings would make the program look good in a year-end report. However, now you are more aware of the response bias inherent in client-satisfaction surveys, namely that respondents tend to report high satisfaction ratings, particularly for the instructor and the program overall. You are concerned about the mixed reactions to particular features of the program. For instance, 35 percent were extremely or moderately dissatisfied with the exercises themselves. Was it the skill level required? The pace? The type of exercise? Over half the respondents were dissatisfied with the facilities, 46 percent with the schedule, and 42 percent with the location. Why were these people dissatisfied?

In particular, be wary of using general yes or no questions concerning perceived benefits as an indicator of outcome (as shown at the bottom of table 3.2). In chapter 4, I discuss in more detail how retrospective reports are not highly credible and why you need to compare baseline assessments with assessments following participation to examine client outcomes.

As discussed above, such numerical ratings do not tell you why people were satisfied or dissatisfied. Thus, some client-satisfaction forms also include open-ended questions to obtain more detailed feedback. Typical open-ended questions are as follows:

What did you like most *about the program?*

What did you like least *about the program?*

If you could change one thing about this program, what would it be?

Do you have any comments or suggestions to help us improve the program?

So, what do you do with these open-ended comments? First, report the response rate for each question (how many of those who received the survey answered these items or provided comments?). People often leave these blank because they do not want to bother filling them out, or because they are reluctant to be too specific due to fear of being identified. Remember that the positivity bias applies to open-ended, as well as to forced-choice ratings. Criticisms, when they do appear, are more likely to target program features

than the service provider. Chapter 7 shows you how to do a systematic content analysis of such nonnumerical data. Most programs simply read through the batch of comments provided.

You may find contradictions: the things some people most like about the program are the same as those others most dislike (music selection, for example). Sometimes, one or two objections will stand out. For instance, several people may complain that the music is too loud or class time is too long or scheduled too late in the day. If you get specific comments, and the same comments repeatedly, you have some potentially useful information.

Ideally, you want to know which types of participants are more or less satisfied with various aspects of your program. For instance, is the location inconvenient for people who use public transportation to get to the program? Are retirees more dissatisfied with the current class schedule? Is the scheduling of the class meeting the needs of people with young children or those who work? What would they prefer? As you can see, the results of client-satisfaction surveys alone are often not informative. Because such surveys tend to be anonymous, you have no way of linking the responses to other sources of information, such as characteristics of respondents. You also cannot link these response patterns to patterns of attendance or usage. Are the people who are the most dissatisfied with program location or schedule attending less often?

To obtain such information, client-satisfaction questionnaires sometimes include a section asking respondents to provide some basic information about themselves, such as gender and age. Such surveys could also include a question on frequency of attendance. Keep in mind that if the class is small, participants may be unwilling to supply such personal information because they could easily be identified. For instance, if there are only a few males in the class, gender would be an easy identifier. The reason client surveys are anonymous in the first place is to protect confidentiality and encourage honest responses, particularly concerning ratings of the service providers or program instructors.

There are alternatives to satisfaction surveys. Comment cards and suggestion boxes present an opportunity for disgruntled clients to express their views before they leave the program—often before the program- or year-end survey. Grantham et al. (1998) recommend exit interviews to find out why people are leaving.

> **Y**ou can also obtain client feedback through comment cards, suggestion boxes, personal or telephone interviews, and focus groups.

Another strategy is to implement a standard procedure for contacting absent participants, hopefully before they become complete dropouts. Chapter 6 contains an example of such a structured telephone interview. Structured interviews of absent members can provide feedback to the program as well as being a motivational technique to encourage potential dropouts to return to the program.

I also highly recommend holding focus groups with clients, particularly when you need to make major decisions (for instance, purchasing different types of fitness equipment, expanding a clubhouse, starting a new line of programming). Such discussions will generate far more detailed and insightful feedback than survey questionnaires. Later chapters will show you when and how to conduct focus groups.

Summary

Programs frequently do not make full use of the information at their disposal. Total head counts of new and former members and aggregate usage rates are the norm. Much information is collected from individual clients but not used to develop profiles across clients. Evaluation can help you customize your information system by collecting only the information you need, in the form you need it, to guide program decision making.

The chapter provided simple formulas for determining membership growth, attrition, and duration. First, however, you need to record individual attendance or usage patterns. It is also easy to develop profiles of your continuing and discontinuing clients by collecting more detailed information as new clients join your facility or register for your program. You may also use some information you currently collect (and put in client folders) in this regard.

This chapter provided examples of customizing formulas to calculate dropout rate based on the length of a given program session. The remainder of the book will help you customize each type of information you collect.

The beauty of a client-information system is that you can learn a great deal about dropout patterns and characteristics without ever having to contact or speak to the dropouts themselves! By obtaining a comprehensive client profile at intake and tracking individual participation rates, your client-information system can tell you about characteristics of frequent versus infrequent users, and those of continuing versus discontinuing clients. However, you still need to examine reasons for leaving to modify features of program accessibility or delivery under your control.

Although client-satisfaction surveys are popular, be aware of their limitations. You can expect a positive response bias, particularly concerning ratings of the service deliverer. Such surveys also tend to underrepresent infrequent attendees and miss program dropouts. Numerical or forced-choice ratings—whether excellence, satisfaction, or thumbs up—are difficult to interpret. Specific comments to open-ended questions may be more enlightening, but be careful not to act too quickly on a few comments without investigating further. This does not mean that you should do away with client-satisfaction surveys, but you should consider supplementing such surveys with other strategies for soliciting input of current and former clients.

Working Exercises

1. List the types of information you routinely obtain from your clients. Consider how you currently use this information.

2. If someone asked you to describe the clients in each of your programs and across your facility, how much detail could you provide? How confident are you that this data is accurate?

3. How many new clients do you get monthly and annually? How many clients leave over the same periods?

4. What criteria do you use to determine program absence and dropout?

5. How do you record attendance, participation, or usage rates? Do you do this for each client in each class or program?

6. Do you currently conduct client-satisfaction surveys; if so, how often? What do you do with the information you obtain from such surveys? Do you consider the response rate?

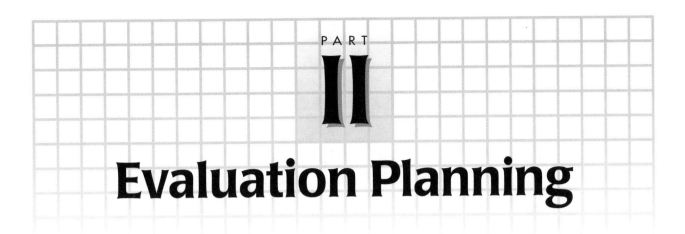

PART

II

Evaluation Planning

The first part of this book presents reasons why all exercise leaders should consider doing program evaluation—regardless of the sector they work in, the type of clientele they work with, or the type of exercise service they provide. For each scenario in chapter 1, I suggested specific types of evaluation (e.g., needs assessment or outcome evaluation) based on the issues raised by the exercise leaders. This part of the book explains precisely what each type of evaluation involves.

You know from chapter 2 the importance of marketing your exercise services to recruit new clients; you address market analysis and testing through needs assessment and formative evaluation, respectively. You also know that to optimize service delivery, you need to examine patterns of usage and dropout, potential barriers to participation, as well as client satisfaction. You address these issues through process evaluation. Outcome evaluation, meanwhile, allows you to examine the extent to which your clients are benefiting from participation.

Part II deals with evaluation planning. Chapter 4 explains and illustrates the differences among various types of evaluation: needs assessment, formative evaluation, implementation evaluation, process evaluation, outcome evaluation, and cost analysis. As part of the planning

process, you will also learn how to develop clear program objectives and establish realistic targets for demonstrating program performance. Chapter 4 will help you prioritize your evaluation activities by focusing on those that are the most relevant, timely, and practical for your program.

Chapter 5 helps you select your evaluation tools. I review the pros and cons of various data-collection options—existing records, observation, questionnaires, telephone surveys, interviews, and focus groups—in terms of feasibility from the program's perspective, acceptability from your clients' perspective, and credibility from other stakeholders' perspective. By learning what is involved in developing and administering various measures, you will be able to make informed choices and justify your methods to other stakeholders. Although programs need to develop some of their own measures, such as client-background questionnaires, a wide variety of published and credible tools are available for outcome evaluation. Chapter 5 shows you several examples of physical and psychological measures to assess client benefits and concludes by recommending the data-collection strategies that are most practical for programs undertaking their own needs assessment, formative, implementation, process, or outcome evaluation.

Focusing Your Evaluation Activities

By now you realize that there are several approaches to evaluation, such as needs assessment, process evaluation, and outcome evaluation. This chapter explains and illustrates what each approach involves to help you select the most relevant approach for your program. As part of the planning process, you will learn how to develop clear program objectives and establish realistic targets for demonstrating program performance. By the end of this chapter you will be able to focus your activities and prioritize your evaluation projects.

The preface opened with a simple definition of program evaluation—the process of collecting and using information to guide decision making. Now I will elaborate on this definition.

> **P**rogram evaluation is the systematic process of collecting credible information for timely decision making about implementing, operating, modifying, continuing, or expanding a program.

This more formal definition describes the types of decisions that evaluation can guide. This definition also encompasses the various approaches to program evaluation: needs assessment, formative evaluation, implementation evaluation, process evaluation, outcome evaluation, and cost analysis. Although the purpose of each approach differs, all share the following features: systematic collection of credible information for timely program decision making.

By *systematic*, I mean that there is a clear purpose or rationale for why you are collecting the information, with the end use and the intended users of the information in mind. You need to be confident that you are using the right approach to obtain the kinds of information you want. *Credibility* is particularly important if you intend to share the evaluation plan and findings with other stakeholders. Finally, evaluation must be *timely*. A project that takes two years to complete may not be in the best interests of a program that needs to make decisions about continuation or expansion today (or more likely yesterday). What you most need to know and when are key considerations in prioritizing your evaluation activities.

> **I** was first contacted by the Canadian Red Cross Society's Fun & Fitness Program to assist with evaluation in the spring of 1982. The program's coordinator realized that believing in their program was not enough. They needed ammunition to support the program and needed this ammunition quickly, because the board had scheduled a major review of all their community programs in four months. Given the time line, and the fact that few new groups were starting over the summer months, we decided to postpone the outcome evaluation and conduct a process evaluation that summer. Evidence of high demand, participation, and satisfaction was credible and timely for these policy makers. In fact, Fun & Fitness received accolades because it was one of the few community services under review that provided any evaluation evidence. Fun & Fitness was spared the axe; other programs were not as fortunate. Moreover, we used the evaluation findings to justify additional funds for training more instructors (Myers and Hamilton 1985).

Your program's development stage is the best gauge for deciding which evaluation approach is the most appropriate and timely. For example, the Fun & Fitness Program had been operating for several years before considering evaluation. When a program is up and running, process and outcome evaluation are the most relevant types of evaluation to consider. For several reasons, this program chose to do process evaluation first. The next section takes you through each type of evaluation based on stage of program development. Refer to table 4.1 as we examine each approach.

Needs Assessment

Recall that chapter 2 discussed strategic targeting of exercise programs and services. You should conduct needs assessments (also called market analyses) in the initial planning or idea stage to help make the decisions of whether to offer a new program or service, to whom, and how.

> **N**eeds assessment is the systematic appraisal of the type and scope of an unmet need, the characteristics and preferences of the intended target group, and the nature and scope of existing services directed at this target group.

You usually need a rationale when applying for funding or otherwise justifying a new program to internal or external stakeholders. This rationale should include evidence that the service in question is needed, wanted, and not currently being offered in the area (or at least the market is not saturated or overserviced). Typically, the proposal also includes a description of the intended target audience, proposed activities, and projected resources. Table 4.1 describes the generic questions that needs assessment addresses and the four sources of information typically used to answer these questions.

Demographic, Social, and Health Indicators

Commercial markets would never launch a new product without first knowing the size of their intended target audience. Demographic indicators tell you about the size and distribution of the population residing in your area. For instance, how many young adults (age 18 to 29) live in the area? What is the proportion of males to females?

Programs may also be interested in other characteristics of the population in their area. Social indicators are calculated based on several demographic characteristics. Examples of social indicators are ethnicity (based on ancestry, country of birth, languages spoken), household composition (based on number of dwellers and relationships between dwellers), household income (based on number of earners), and job classifications (based on education, position, type of occupation, and earnings). Similarly, unemployment, poverty, and divorce rates are social indicators based on several factors. Health indicators, meanwhile, tell you about the prevalence of certain health problems in your surrounding region, such as the number of people with heart disease, osteoporosis, or diabetes, and the health-related behaviors of the population in the area, such as the number of smokers.

Demographic, social, and health indicators are often used to justify public health and clinical programs. For example, recall scenario 2 (p. 7) on the textile plant wellness program. The health educator had data for the region showing a high prevalence of smoking, obesity, and physical inactivity. She also knew the demographic and social profile of the community—primarily young, blue-collar workers with families. Based on these indicators, she could make an argument that her community, particularly the women, had unmet physical activity needs.

Existing Services

In addition to investigating the profile of potential consumers, commercial marketers always check the competition in the area—who else is selling a similar product or service? The business section of telephone directories and the classified sections of local newspapers can assist entrepreneurs in this regard. For instance, how many multipurpose fitness clubs are offered in the area? How many personal trainers are advertising their services? How many clinics offer sports medicine and rehabilitation services?

Table 4.1 Linking Evaluation Approach to Stage of Program Development

Program stage	Types of questions	Type of evaluation	Information sources
Initial planning	What is the rationale for the program? Who is the intended audience? What is the need and demand? Do such services already exist in the area? How to advertise? Projected activities? Projected resources?	Needs assessment Market analysis	Demographic, social, and health indicators Existing services Key informants Potential clients
Development	How does the target group respond?	Formative evaluation Market testing	Target audience
Early implementation	According to plan?	Implementation evaluation	Site visits Records or invoices Minutes of meetings
Routine operation	What is the usage level or participation rate? How many go through the program, at what intervals? Who discontinues? What are the barriers to use? What are delivery constraints?	Process evaluation	Program records Current clients Dropouts Workload analysis
Stable operation (at least one year)	What are the effects of participation? Are there negative or adverse effects? What percentage of clients improve (maintain), how much, and over what period? Which clients benefit most?	Outcome evaluation	New clients assessed at entry and at follow-up
Further planning	Should we consider new targets? Is the target group aware of the service? Do competing services now exist?	Periodic needs assessment	Demographic, social, and health indicators Existing services Key informants Potential clients
Initial planning development Stable operation	What are the costs of the various inputs (advertising, overhead, staffing, equipment)? What is the cost per case? What is the cost to produce various client outcomes?	Cost analysis	Projected costs Development costs Operational costs Case analysis Cost-outcome analysis

It is also important for nonprofit agencies, health promoters, and recreational planners to check whether similar programs are available in their area before implementing a possibly redundant service. Find out what services already exist and which populations they serve. Directories may be of initial assistance to identify such services, but you will likely have to contact key informants to obtain more detailed information on the nature of their services and their clientele.

> **B**efore we launch any new programs or instructor-training initiatives at the Centre for Activity and Ageing, we first check out what services are already available in our area. Using a provincial directory of nursing homes, it was simple to determine that 27 such facilities were located in our region. To determine whether they currently offered exercise programs, however, we needed to contact the administrator of each facility. We found that most (98 percent) of these facilities said they did offer exercise programs. The next step was to find out more about these exercise programs. With the permission of the administrators, we contacted the recreation director at each facility and conducted a telephone survey. We also visited several facilities to observe their exercise classes. We found that chair-based exercise classes were the norm. Only about a third of the facilities offered any weight-bearing exercises, even though all had ambulatory residents. Moreover, participation rates were low—only 15 percent of residents took part in these exercise classes. Class offerings ranged from three times a week in some facilities to only once a month in others. Limited funds, lack of training, diversity of residents, and challenges in motivating residents were cited as the primary barriers to exercise programming. The findings of this needs assessment provided the rationale for developing the Functional Fitness Long-Term Care (FFLTC) Program and instructor training for nursing home staff (Lazowski et al. in press).

Key Informants

Key informants are the individuals or groups most likely to know about the services being offered to particular groups in the area. For instance, in the example concerning existing exercise programming in nursing homes, facility administrators and recreation directors were our key informants. You can identify key informants for many types of exercise services. Particularly in smaller communities, it is easy to find out who delivers specialized exercise programming such as cardiac rehabilitation. Local chapters of societies for diabetes, stroke, osteoporosis, Alzheimer's, and so on, frequently know what services are available in the area for these populations or can refer you to people who do know. If you are considering targeting seniors in your region, contact your local senior's centers to see what types of programs are available to this group.

A sampling strategy called *snowballing* works well for identifying key informants. People working in a particular area tend to know one another. Physicians know other physicians, physical therapists know other physical therapists, personal trainers know other personal trainers, and so on. Key informants will refer you to colleagues or others working in the same area.

Key informants are a useful source of information concerning the nature of existing services for particular target groups: What's currently available? How do they advertise? Who is using these services? What additional services do they think are needed in the area? Which populations are being underserved? Is there an unmet need?

Potential Clients

Let's say you have established that there is a sufficient market of potential clients, similar services are not being provided in the area, and key informants feel there is a *need* for the new program or service. You still should not make the leap and assume that there is a *demand* for the program or service. Once you decide on your intended target audience, the next step is to find out whether they want the new program or service and under what conditions, such as location, scheduling, and payment plans.

Although the health educator in scenario 2 (p. 7) had evidence that many adults in the community were sedentary, she wanted to know whether the intended target group (blue-collar women in the textile plant) would be interested in the Time for Me wellness program. In scenario 3 (p. 7), the YMCA manager had received a few requests for a Tai Chi program, but he thought it prudent to survey his membership to determine the level of interest in such a program.

Thus, you should consider four sources of information for needs assessment. Demographic, social, and health statistics on the population in your area likely already exist, and you can obtain them from public libraries and health boards. You can use telephone, service directories, and newspaper ads to identify existing services. Key informants and potential clients, however, are critical for learning more about the perceived need and demand for new services in the area. Chapter 5 describes various options for collecting information from these sources.

Many programs, unfortunately, proceed with program implementation without first conducting a needs assessment (Myers 1988), but it is never too late. Even operational programs should consider a needs assessment to check out their competition in the area and to assess demand if they wish to attract more clients (refer to the section on further planning in table 4.1).

Periodic needs assessment is the systematic appraisal (or reappraisal) of consumer awareness, an examination (or reexamination) of whether other similar services are available in the area, and consideration of new markets or target groups.

Given that competing fitness services are continually emerging, it is particularly important that programs considering expansion conduct periodic needs assessments. For instance, you may have had the only exercise program tailored specifically to seniors in your community 10 years ago, but that is unlikely to be the case today. There is also danger in obtaining information only from current members. Let's say a fitness club thought older members might prefer '50s music and age-segregated classes. They surveyed their current members over age 65 and found that they enjoyed participating with younger adults and liked rock music—providing support for current programming. Had they surveyed other older adults in their community, however, they may have discovered a market that would be attracted to classes tailored to their age group. Programs may also discover that some potential consumers were not even aware of their services—they may have to revise their advertising strategies.

As table 4.1 shows, periodic needs assessment involves the same types of information sources as traditional needs assessment; the purpose is still to guide planning and marketing. The only difference is that the application is for ongoing or further planning rather than for initial planning. Depending on the nature of your service and your market, consider periodic needs assessments every 5 to 10 years (Myers 1988).

Formative Evaluation

A needs assessment or market analysis tells you the size of the potential market and whether potential consumers have any interest in the new product or service.

Use this information to justify the costs in developing a new service or targeting a new market. Before you proceed full steam ahead, however, it is wise to conduct a formative evaluation (also referred to as market testing, field testing, or pilot testing). Figure 4.1 helps you visualize this step, which falls between initial planning and putting the program in place.

Formative evaluation is the systematic appraisal of prototype promotional and delivery strategies in the development or draft stage, before full-scale production, distribution, or implementation.

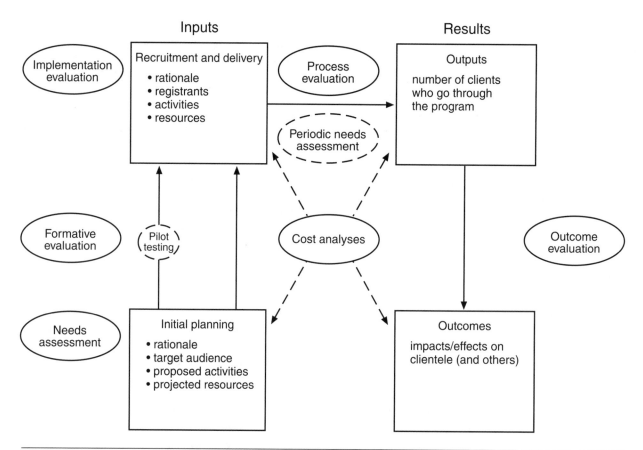

Figure 4.1 Model for focusing evaluation activites.

Adapted, by permission, from J. Hudson, J. Mayne, and R. Thomlison, eds., 1992, Action-oriented evaluation in organizations: Canadian practices. (Toronto: Wall & Emerson), 3. Copyright 1992 by Wall & Emerson, Inc.

Commercial marketers never launch a new product before thoroughly market testing every aspect—pricing, packaging, labeling, and content. Many of us have nibbled our way through the supermarket tasting free samples of new products that may or may not later make it to the shelves. We have seen pilots for TV shows—some of which become long-running series and others that get canned. Consumer feedback is a major factor in deciding whether to launch a new product, whether changes are needed, or whether to go back to the drawing board.

Health promoters are adopting similar strategies when producing educational films, videos, and pamphlets (cf. U.S. Department of Health and Human Services 1992, *Making Health Communication Programs Work: A Planner's Guide*). One particular concern of health educators is that their target audience understands their messages. They often subject printed materials (i.e., brochures, pamphlets, and booklets) to readability analysis in the draft stage. You can use simple formulas (described in the aforementioned planner's guide, as

well as in Fry 1977 and McLaughlin 1969) to examine the complexity of printed messages and estimate the school grade equivalent required to read the material. You can then compare this finding with the educational level of the intended target audience and simplify the printed material if necessary.

Although they can provide you with usable information, readability assessments alone are an insufficient indicator of comprehension and do not tell you anything about whether messages are appealing or convincing. Focus groups or other strategies for obtaining feedback from the intended target group are still necessary to explore these issues.

For instance, the health educator in scenario 2 (p. 7) might hold focus groups with women from the textile plant to get their reactions to the proposed program title (Time for Me) and their input on delivery and scheduling options. Program titles or slogans can be powerful in turning potential consumers on or off. This is why commercial marketers spend a great deal of time market testing product packaging and labeling.

*W*hen our Centre for Activity and Ageing was developing our Home Support Exercise Program, we obtained reactions from a sample of home care workers and clients who were asked to try out the new instructional video, booklet, and exercises. Based on their feedback, we changed all three components. For instance, one exercise (the braid walk) was found to be too difficult for some clients, so we deleted this exercise and modified the instructional booklet accordingly. Our sample also suggested using more ethnic models and older adults at various levels of ability in the video, so we revised the video. Given the high costs involved in production and distribution, particularly the video, the time and money spent in the formative or development stage was well worth the effort to make the program more acceptable for its intended audience.

Implementation Evaluation

Once you have made the decision to proceed with the new program or service, you need to monitor whether things are going according to plan via implementation evaluation. You may need to build or renovate facilities; hire and train staff; put advertising into place; purchase equipment; produce pamphlets, posters, or videos; and so forth.

*I*mplementation evaluation is the systematic appraisal of the extent to which a program or service conforms to the original plan.

For instance, in scenario 4 (p. 7), the manager needs to determine whether the active living posters were produced. Were the posters put up in the three targeted malls? When? Were the posters still there a week later (or were they ripped down or defaced)?

As table 4.1 shows, site visits or observations; records, such as purchase invoices; and minutes

of planning meetings are the most common sources of information used for implementation evaluation. Implementation evaluation is a straightforward process of monitoring to ensure that program components and activities are being put into place and to determine whether this has occurred on schedule, ahead of schedule, or behind schedule.

Process Evaluation

Once the program is up and running—staff have been hired, clients are registered, classes are being offered, and equipment has arrived—it is time to do process evaluation.

*P*rocess evaluation is the systematic appraisal of program delivery and usage under routine or normal operation.

Table 4.1 shows the generic questions addressed through process evaluation. These types of questions should sound familiar, because I raised them in chapter 2 (concerning factors affecting adoption and adherence) and in chapter 3 (concerning client-information systems). The distinction between process evaluation and ongoing program monitoring has become increasingly blurred as organizations develop more sophisticated client- and management-information systems (Rossi, Freeman, and Lipsey 1999).

If you already have a good record-keeping system, some of the information you need to monitor your operations, such as staffing and delivery patterns and usage rates, may be readily available for quarterly, semiannual, or annual reports. However, most programs usually need to collect additional information, such as perceived barriers, for process evaluation purposes. As described in chapter 3, many programs do not have a detailed enough profile of their clientele to determine whether they are reaching their intended target audience (see cartoon, p. 48).

For example, the intended target audience of the low-intensity Fun & Fitness program was fairly healthy, but sedentary, older adults. Our process evaluation revealed that actual participants ranged from the frail to the highly active senior. Even though the program and leadership

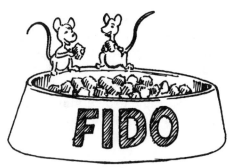

Intended target audience
versus actual users

training were not designed for frail, institutionalized persons, lack of available exercise programming for this population (particularly in the early 1980s) led recreation directors to adopt the Fun & Fitness model. At the other extreme, we found one class in which many participants jogged or biked miles to get to and from this low-intensity class! Their instructor did not believe Fun & Fitness was meeting their physical activity needs, but training and liability concerns precluded offering a more advanced exercise program. These findings led the Red Cross to reexamine the program's training, promotion, and screening procedures (Myers and Hamilton 1985).

A more complex example is a process evaluation of a multifaceted health promotion program delivered to businesses through a mobile van called the HeartMobile. The objectives of the HeartMobile are to increase awareness of heart disease risk factors and to promote healthier lifestyles through smoking cessation, stress management, increased physical activity, weight loss, and dietary modifications. A 20-minute tour through the van involves health-risk screening and modular presentations. As they leave, participants receive a passport summarizing their personalized computer-scored health-risk assessment, blood pressure readings, cholesterol level, and body mass index zone.

The deliverers—a public health unit—routinely recorded the number of requests, the number and type of businesses who receive the program, and the number of employees who go through the program at each work site. The health unit also had copies of each participating company's summary profile of employee health-risk appraisals. Despite all their routinely collected records, after four years of operation the program felt they could benefit from conducting a formal process

evaluation. We held six focus groups in different work sites: three with blue-collar employees and three with white-collar employees (managerial level) who had gone through the HeartMobile. In a nutshell, we found that some modules were perceived as more useful than others. For instance, some participants felt that they learned little new information through the smoking module. The evaluation also indicated that blue- and white-collar employees had different needs (e.g., concerning stress management and recreational physical activity). The passport and summary were too difficult for many blue-collar employees (determined by a readability analysis, indicating that the material was at a grade 9 to 11 reading level, and feedback from the focus groups), and some ethnic groups needed translation. Employees on shift work were not being accommodated through current scheduling. Blood testing made some participants feel anxious, and the program label HeartMobile mislead some into thinking diagnostic assessments for heart disease, such as angiocardiograms, would be involved (Gray and Myers 1997).

One lesson to learn from the HeartMobile example is that if this program had conducted formative evaluation or pilot testing before full-scale implementation, they might have saved themselves a great deal of money that they now had to spend revising the expensive logo embossed on the van (viewed as misleading) and the passport (viewed as too difficult).

Another lesson from both examples is that you could not obtain this information through program records alone. By the same token, it would not be economical to collect all this information on an ongoing basis. You need to carry out process evaluations to obtain in-depth feedback from clients only periodically. Specific and timely evaluation projects to address key issues as they arise, such as whether members want a Tai Chi program or a swimming pool, are often more useful than annually handing out general client-satisfaction surveys to everyone.

Many scenarios presented in chapter 1 could benefit from doing process evaluation. For example, in scenario 1 (p. 6) the corporate fitness program wanted to know why only 20 percent of employees tried the aerobics class, and why half of these stopped coming. Because this company has its own on-site exercise studio, they might also want to know which pieces of equipment their employees use most and whether they would prefer (and more likely use) different equipment or types of classes. Through process evaluation, the program might find that some employees prefer to play team sports, others prefer to work out on their own (and want more treadmills in the exercise room), and some who prefer the exercise classes at noon or in the morning before work (as opposed to 4:30).

In scenario 6 (p. 8), the recreation director in the nursing home wanted to demonstrate not only the therapeutic benefits, but also the *feasibility* of challenging exercise classes. Process evaluation addresses the latter. We conducted an evaluation of a similar model—the Functional Fitness for Long-Term Care (FFLTC) program—in four LTC facilities (Lazowski et al. in press). We found that training one staff member, who in turn trained other staff and volunteers, was an economical way of delivering the program. Low-cost, portable materials, such as resistance bands and soft weights, reduced equipment costs. By providing supervision, assistance with standing, and chair backs for support, even residents considered nonambulatory were able to perform the exercises. For lower functioning residents and those with cognitive impairments, smaller classes of three to five participants or more volunteers to assist the instructor were needed. For higher functioning residents with greater mobility, a 10:1 client-to-instructor ratio was possible (Lazowski et al. in press).

In scenario 7 (p. 9), the diabetes self-management program, the manager was interested in examining program delivery, specifically educational messages concerning physical activity. My colleagues and I have conducted a process evaluation of such a diabetes education program (Tudor-Locke et al. 1998). We found that diabetes educators knew how to counsel their clients about nutrition and weight loss but were unsure how to advise them concerning exercise. Clients, not surprisingly, were receiving unclear and often conflicting messages. We used interviews with a sample of diabetes educators, and focus groups with samples of clients, to conduct this process evaluation.

You can collect process evaluation information simultaneously with outcome evaluation. Ideally, however, you carry out process evaluations *before* outcome evaluations. The reasoning for this sequence is that process evaluation findings often reveal areas in which you can improve program delivery. When such factors are under your control and you can address them with available resources, it is highly preferable to first act on the findings of process evaluation and modify your program accordingly before conducting outcome evaluation. You want to examine the benefits of your program under the best possible delivery conditions.

Outcome Evaluation

Table 4.1 illustrates the types of questions that you can address through outcome evaluation. Outcome evaluation addresses the bottom line— is the program effective? Does the program make a difference in clients' lives? Are clients any different or better than they would have been without the program or service?

> **O***utcome evaluation* is the systematic appraisal of the program's impact on clients, in relation to level of program participation and baseline characteristics. Outcome evaluation, summative evaluation, and impact evaluation are interchangeable terms.

For many programs, the intended or desired outcome is improvement or positive change (e.g., increase in physical fitness, decrease in pain). For other programs, the intended outcome may be maintaining functional ability, such as mobility; physical status, such as body weight or nonsmoking status; or behavior (e.g., sustaining regular exercise patterns). Still other programs may be prevention oriented (e.g., preventing further heart attacks through cardiac rehabilitation, preventing further work-related injuries, preventing diabetes-related complications). Thus, program impact or benefits of participation may refer to improvement, maintenance, or prevention.

It is also important to keep in mind that interventions may potentially have negative or adverse effects on clients. For instance, if the program promotes weight loss, clients who do not lose weight, or not as much as they would like, may experience frustration and decreased self-esteem. Exercise-related injuries are obvious adverse effects all programs should consider. When planning outcome evaluations, it is important to consider the possible adverse effects as well as the positive benefits of participation—in other words, the total impacts of the program.

Do not conduct outcome evaluation prematurely. The next section addresses issues of timing and credibility in planning outcome evaluation projects and shows you a sequential or staged approach for evaluating your programs in manageable pieces.

Timing

Most programs go through a shakedown or settling period, in which they make refinements to staffing and delivery patterns, such as scheduling or program content. As noted in the previous section, process evaluation can provide direction on what is working well and what you can improve or modify through shifting available resources. For instance, more classes might be indicated for peak periods and fewer classes for low periods. You may revise program materials so they are easier to understand or more appealing for clients, or you may address overcrowding and pacing considerations.

Once your program is stable—in staffing and delivery patterns—you are ready to plan for outcome evaluation. The stabilization period will vary from program to program, and each program will need to make this determination. As a rule, programs should be fully operational for at least a year before doing outcome evaluation (refer to table 4.1).

Credibility

As noted in chapter 3 regarding client-satisfaction surveys, programs should be wary of simply asking clients whether they feel they have benefited from the program or service. Personal testimonials are not highly credible for several reasons.

First, there is the problem of memory or retrospective reporting bias (people may have difficulty accurately remembering what they were like before the program). Second, there is the assumption that clients would not have changed, improved, or maintained without the intervention. In some cases, this assumption may be correct. For instance, without exercise, we can expect frail, older adults (as in scenario 6, p. 8) to show decrements in mobility, balance, and

strength (Lazowski et al. in press). Conversely, we know that people with low-back pain following injury (as in scenario 5, p. 8) will spontaneously improve over time whether they are treated or not (cf. Williams and Myers 1998a). Third, personal testimonials are vulnerable to attention bias. Some people may say they have benefited or improved simply because they like the program deliverers and want to please them.

As chapter 5 shows, you can use personal testimonials (e.g., quotes from satisfied participants) for identifying which types of outcomes clients perceive to be personally relevant to help you choose meaningful indicators and measures. As chapter 7 discusses, personal testimonials are also useful to enliven an evaluation report. Outcome evaluations based solely on anecdotes and testimonials, however, are unlikely to be seen as highly credible.

As the following examples illustrate, programs need to systematically assess clients *before* they begin participation (at entry or baseline) and *after* some period of participation (at follow-up) to examine program impacts (improvement, maintenance, or prevention).

Earlier in this chapter (see p. 48), I presented some results of the HeartMobile's process evaluation. The intended outcomes of this work site health promotion program are to increase knowledge of cardiovascular risk factors and to promote changes in related behaviors. The outcome evaluation of this program used questionnaires to measure changes in knowledge and lifestyle practices (diet, physical activity, etc.). We assessed a sample of participants before going through the program, and again six weeks following participation (Gray and Myers 1997). We found that participants were already knowledgeable about some risk factors (e.g., smoking) at pretest, and the program made little impact on their knowledge in this area. Positive change, however, was found in other areas of knowledge and lifestyle practices, such as physical activity and diet, as shown by increased scores on the questionnaire measures.

In the outcome evaluation of FFLTC, we compared residents who received this program over a four-month period with residents who received a less challenging program (a seated, range-of-motion, or ROM, class) over the same period. Both classes were group based and run by trained staff members for 45 minutes, three times per week. Assessments at baseline and at four months consisted of mobility, balance, gait, flexibility, functional capacity, and several measures of strength (Lazowski et al. in press). Four months of exercise led to significant improvements in mobility (16 percent average change), balance (9 percent), flexibility (36 percent), and knee (55 percent) and hip (12 percent) strength for the FFLTC group. Shoulder strength was the only improvement found for the ROM group. The latter group deteriorated over the four-month period in some areas, particularly hip strength, mobility, and functional ability (Lazowski et al. in press). This outcome study not only provided dramatic support for the more challenging, total-body conditioning program for frail, institutionalized residents, but also demonstrated clear benefits over the status quo or typical, seated exercise programming.

Given the resources and expertise available at our university-affiliated Centre for Activity and Ageing, we were able to administer multiple measures of client outcomes and compare the relative effectiveness of two programs. It is highly unlikely that the recreation director in scenario 6 (see p. 8), however, would be able to conduct such an elaborate outcome evaluation. It is more likely that she would conduct a modest and feasible outcome evaluation by selecting only a few key measures, such as mobility, assessing participants before and after participation, and using a simple formula to calculate percent improvement (see chapter 7).

Taking a Sequential Approach

If you are planning the first outcome evaluation of your program, consider a sequential or staged approach. For instance, don't worry about comparing the relative effectiveness of your different classes or programs until you have tackled one class or program at a time. Don't worry about demonstrating long-term outcomes, such as maintaining body weight, until you have examined short-term effects, such as weight loss.

Using weight loss as a simple example, let's look at a sequential approach to examining outcomes. Remember that you need to look at new clients, people who have just entered your program. Continuing clients may already have changed as a result of participation. As a first step, measure the weight (or girth or body mass index [BMI])of new clients. Then, reassess these people

after a reasonable time in the program. Essentially what you are doing is tracking a sample of your clients. If you find that none, or few, are losing weight, then you need to go back to the drawing board and think about why. It may be that clients are not complying with the regimen (e.g., they may be increasing energy expenditure but not decreasing energy or caloric intake). It may also be that either the type or amount of exercise is insufficient for weight loss. Program modifications may be in order before you proceed further with examining client outcomes.

On the other hand, if you find that some clients have lost weight, then you should proceed to document the proportion losing weight and the amount of weight lost. Next, you want to know which types of clients lose more weight than others. You also want to examine whether weight loss is related to class attendance or participation rate.

The point is that you can approach outcome evaluation in stages or manageable chunks. You can also save yourself time and effort by not prematurely collecting information. Part III provides details on when and how to collect outcome data, how to calculate change, and how to link information (client change, characteristics, and participation rates).

Cost Analysis

Outcome evaluation addresses program *effectiveness;* cost analysis addresses program *efficiency.* As both figure 4.1 and table 4.1 show, cost analysis applies to various stages of program development. In the initial planning stage, programs must estimate or project the cost of resources required to deliver a given service. In the development stage, programs incur capital costs, such as equipment purchases and advertising costs. Once they are up and running, programs have direct operating expenses, such as salaries and benefits, and indirect expenses, such as custodial services and overhead. Most programs closely monitor fiscal revenues and expenditures for audit purposes.

*C*ost analysis or efficiency evaluation is the systematic appraisal of program costs in relation to program results.

There are several types of cost analysis. For instance, you might want to examine the cost-effectiveness of your advertisement or recruitment strategies by calculating the average cost for attracting a new member. The term *relative cost-effectiveness* suggests comparison, such as the number of new members attracted through radio versus newspaper ads or the number of new members in the current year compared with the previous year.

You can use crude calculations (total program costs divided by total number of participants over a given period) to estimate the average service cost per case. Such calculations may be of more interest to clinical exercise programs than to commercial facilities. For instance, workers compensation (or other insurers) want to know the average cost for treating injured workers or accident victims through rehabilitation clinics.

Some programs may be able to quantify client benefits and relate these to service costs. *Cost-benefit analysis* has been conducted for industrial fitness programs. In cost-benefit analysis, you must calculate costs from both the program's perspective and participants' perspective, such as fees, transportation, baby-sitting, time off work. Similarly, you must translate societal benefits (e.g., savings for the employer or for workers compensation) and client benefits (e.g., recovery) into monetary terms. As you can appreciate, this is not a simple matter. What is the dollar value for reduced suffering or improved well-being?

Browne (1984) reported reductions of 46 percent in medical expenses, 20 percent in number of disability days, and 32 percent in direct disability costs after one year of a work site fitness program. The cost to operate the fitness program (adjusted for inflation) averaged $121 per employee, and combined savings averaged $354 per employee—a dramatic 3:1 benefit-to-cost ratio.

Cost-outcome, also termed *cost-effectiveness analysis*, is a more feasible approach than cost-benefit analysis because you do not need to express the outcome or effectiveness part of the equation in monetary terms. For instance, Hatziandreu (1988) examined the impact of exercise in preventing coronary heart disease (CHD). They estimated that if 1,000 men beginning at age 35 were to exercise three times per week (20 minutes per session) for 30 years, 530 total years would be gained by preventing CHD. This group would spend a total of 522.7 years exercising, resulting in a difference of 7.3 years of increased life expectancy. This study illustrates the significance of relating exercise participation to mortality and morbidity from a population-health perspective. However, their findings translate into a net gain of only 2.7 days of increased life expectancy for each individual. Obviously, exercise must have other, more immediate benefits to sustain the investment of time and energy from an individual perspective.

What public health planners want to know through cost analysis is different from what most exercise programmers need to know. Clinicians are interested in cost-outcome analysis from the perspective of the cost required to produce certain levels of client outcomes, such as managing hypertension, achieving glycemic control in persons with diabetes, getting injured workers back to work, or restoring functioning in stroke victims. Some outcome indicators, such as level of hypertension or glycemic control, are easy to measure, but most are not as straightforward as they first appear. For instance, return to work is regularly recorded by rehabilitation clinics dealing with injured workers, as in scenario 5 (p. 8). Return to work is used as a proxy (or substitute) indicator for client recovery. However, return to work can be influenced by fear of job loss, financial resources, job satisfaction, duty modifications by the employer, and so on (Williams and Myers 1998a).

Sources such as Rossi, Freeman, and Lipsey (1999) provide further information on cost analysis. My intention here was simply to expose you to some issues involved in cost analysis.

*S*chnelle and colleagues (1995) compared the cost outcomes of an exercise intervention for incontinent nursing home residents. It is estimated that over half of this population have problems with urinary incontinence, resulting in substantial costs in staff time, linens, and so on. The high incidence and prevalence of this problem provided a solid justification for the program. Prompted voiding interventions by nursing staff and aids are a common strategy for managing incontinence. Schnelle added an exercise component (sit-to-stands and walking or propelling wheelchairs) to the voiding regimen. Compared with a standard voiding regimen, residents who received the prompted voiding plus exercise had similar decreases in incontinence episodes. However, only the exercise group gained in measures of mobility endurance. The exercise regimen required an additional six minutes of staff time per resident per episode—translating into 18 minutes for a full 8-hour shift. By calculating nursing aids' salary (hourly rate) plus benefits, the additional cost per resident for this regimen worked out to $2.10 per resident per day. Over a four-month period, the cost per resident was estimated at $252 (120 days × $2.10 per day), compared with the estimated services of physical therapist at $1,220 over the same period.

Formulating Program Goals and Objectives

Now you have taken the first step toward focusing your evaluation activities by considering which approach is best suited to your program's stage of development and your needs for information. As part of the evaluation planning process, think about what your program wants to accomplish. The next section looks at program objectives.

*P*rogram goals and objectives are guiding statements of expectations or intentions— what a program hopes to accomplish concerning recruitment, service delivery, outputs, and client outcomes.

Textbooks on evaluation and programs themselves differ in how they use the terms *goals* and *objectives*. Some consider goals as abstract statements (for instance, "to rehabilitate injured workers") and objectives as specific statements that spell out the desired level of accomplishment (for instance, "to return 80 percent of clients to work by three months"). Others use the terms goals and objectives interchangeably, as will this book. Some don't use these terms at all, and refer instead to program aims. For now, forget about how to measure whether you are achieving your program goals, objectives, or aims—we will deal with that issue in the next section. First, it is important to realize that you can generate program objectives at each stage of program planning and development and for each program component, as illustrated in table 4.2.

Recall that when you are proposing a new program or service, you must provide a rationale. Sometimes this rationale takes the form of an overall mission or vision for the program. By definition, mission statements are broad or global. For instance, the YMCA states that their mission is "To put Christian principles into practice through programs that build healthy body, mind, and spirit for all" (YMCA 1995, 7). Such statements are primarily used for public relations purposes or to orient staff on the organization's guiding philosophy but have little utility for evaluation purposes.

The next category—implementation objectives— represents planned or proposed activities that you have not yet put into place. Such objectives (with projected time lines) help keep planning or steering committees on track. Recall, implementation evaluation is used to document the extent to which these proposed activities are carried out. Table 4.2 (p. 55) illustrates several examples of implementation-oriented objective statements.

We examine the third category—service objectives—via process evaluation, for example, Are absentees receiving phone calls? Are printed materials understandable? Is the pace of the exercise class suited to the participants' abilities? To what extent are services being provided? Who is using these services? What are barriers to adoption and adherence?

The next category—output objectives—is statements reflecting the desired results of service promotion and delivery. Membership growth is an example. Service objectives and output objectives are not always easy to distinguish from one another, as illustrated in table 4.2 by the example of consumer satisfaction.

The most important task for programs is to separate service and output objectives from *outcome objectives* (Myers 1996; Patton 1997; Rossi, Freeman, and Lipsey 1999). Programs often get stuck at the level of service and output objectives and fail to formulate client-outcome objectives. Do not assume that just because people buy the exercise video or participate in the exercise program, even if they say they are satisfied with the product or service, that they have benefited in any way.

Figure 4.1 illustrates program inputs versus results. Inputs encompass everything the program does—activities, services, and resources associated with recruitment and delivery. Note that program results comprise two categories—outputs and outcomes. In the business world, outputs refer to the goods and services produced and sold (Hudson, Mayne, and Thomlison 1992). For instance, Ford Motor Company produces and sells cars. The commercial fitness sector sells exercise clothing, equipment, videos, memberships, and other services, such as personal training or massages. In the nonprofit sector, outputs usually consist of the number of people who go through a leisure or clinical program or the number who use the facilities (e.g., the number who use bike or walking trails in parks).

In the business world, production and sales translate into the bottom line—gross earnings. However, sales figures alone tell you nothing about how good the cars or tennis rackets are (how many are returned or need to be recalled). Similarly, just because people are medically treated does not mean they are being discharged from the hospital healthier, or even as healthy as when they entered (they may have complications or acquire infections while in the hospital). We can say the same for rehabilitation programs,

health promotion programs, and all exercise programs and services: *just because individuals go through the program, or receive the service, does not necessarily mean they have benefited.*

Providing fitness classes is a service objective. Achieving a high participation or completion rate may be the associated output objective, and increasing client fitness may be the intended outcome. Providing education is a service-oriented objective. Increasing the number of people going through the program may be the output objective, and increasing knowledge or changing behavior may be the intended client outcomes. Promoting client satisfaction is a service objective; achieving high client satisfaction is an output objective. However, you should never consider client satisfaction as evidence of program impact or outcome.

Finally, note that all the statements in table 4.2 are positive in nature. Program objectives are simply statements of what the program hopes to accomplish (positive intentions). Evaluation is necessary to examine and document the extent to which programs are achieving their intended objectives and whether there are any unintended, adverse effects of participation.

Establishing Performance Indicators and Targets

Today, *performance measurement* and *results-based management* are popular buzzwords in the public sector. Due to rising deficits and decreasing public confidence, programs are being pressured to document results. For instance, in the United States, government agencies are now required to develop strategic plans, revised every three years, to identify performance measures and set annual performance targets for each program (Newcomer 1997; Wholey and Newcomer 1997). Unfortunately, the pressure for results-based performance has led to choosing indicators and targets that look good, are readily available, and are easily quantified, such as high client-satisfaction ratings. Service outputs rather than client outcomes, unfortunately, are often used to demonstrate program performance (Myers 1996; Newcomer 1997).

When applying for funding or otherwise lobbying for a new program, everyone wants to make their proposal look as good as possible. For instance, a program may take general objectives, such as to attract clients and improve health, and make these statements more explicit (for instance,

Table 4.2 Sample Program Objectives

A. Program rationale	**Broad mission statements**
	To promote health and well-being
	To obtain a reasonable return on capital investment
B. Program inputs	**Implementation objectives**
B1. Planning	To strike a planning committee
	To develop a brochure
	To distribute a video
	To orient and train staff and volunteers
	To organize a fitness challenge
	To build a new swimming pool
B2. Recruitment and delivery	**Process (service) objectives**
	To attract new clients
	To obtain more referrals
	To offer a Tai Chi class
	To provide information or education
	To provide opportunity for socialization
	To promote consumer satisfaction
C. Program results	**Output objectives**
C1. Outputs	To achieve a high satisfaction rating
	To increase the rate of program completion
	To increase the number of participants in the fitness challenge
	To reduce the annual attrition rate
	To sell more home exercise videos
	To reduce the cost-to-case ratio
C2. Outcomes	**Client-oriented (outcome) objectives**
	To increase knowledge
	To increase physical activity level
	To increase physical fitness
	To decrease body weight
	To enhance self-esteem, confidence
	To maintain functioning
	To decrease pain
	To prevent complications of diabetes

attract 100 new clients over the next six months, achieve a 20-pound average weight loss in the first six months of participation). This program has now set performance indicators and targets against which to judge their service-oriented and client-oriented objectives, respectively.

Table 4.3 Examples of Performance Objectives, Indicators, Targets, and Benchmarks

	Objective	**Indicator**	**Target**	**Benchmark**
Example 1	To deliver better service	Client-satisfaction ratings	90% moderate to high ratings	80% moderate to high ratings in previous year
Example 2	To decrease annual attrition rate	# of clients lost divided by # of new clients at start of year	25% attrition rate next year	Industry standard of 35% Program's rate of 38% in previous year
Example 3	To improve physical fitness	Assessment of BMI, cardiovascular capacity, strength, flexibility	% improvement over baseline level	Yet to be developed
Example 4	To improve extent of client weight loss	Body weight in pounds (lb)	65% of clients will lose at least 10 lb in six months	50% lost at least 10 lb over six-month period in past year
Example 5	To reduce the rate of reinjury	Worker compensation claims	Fewer than 25% of clients will report subsequent back injuries 12 months following program completion	Reinjury rate averaged 43% over past three years

Performance objectives or *program objectives* are simply statements of what a program hopes to accomplish. *Performance indicators* (also called success criteria or operational indicators) specify evidence of accomplishment. *Performance targets* are specific levels or amounts of intended accomplishment, often over a defined period of time.

Note that some sample objective statements in table 4.2 contained specific indicators, such as "to decrease body weight," and other statements were more general (you still need to develop specific indicators for the objective "to increase physical fitness"). None of the statements in table 4.2, however, contained targets, such as how much weight loss to expect.

Although it is tempting to set ambitious performance targets, keep in mind that your program may be judged against these lofty expectations. If this is the first time you are offering your program, and you have no information on what to expect from such programs, you should *not* set arbitrary performance targets. As Patton (1997) notes, "The best basis for establishing future performance targets is past performance" (p. 162). The one exception concerns implementation objectives in which you must establish schedule and budget projections in advance (for instance, when negotiating with contractors to build a swimming pool).

As mentioned in chapter 2, findings of other programs can serve as possible benchmarks or standards for comparison, provided your activities and clientele are similar. However, the most relevant information for establishing realistic performance targets comes from tracking and documenting your program accomplishments.

Table 4.3 provides five examples of program objectives, indicators, targets, and benchmarks. The first two examples address service-oriented and output objectives; the last three address client-outcome objectives.

Four examples have specific indicators and targets based on either benchmarks from similar programs or documented performance in the programs themselves. Example 3 represents a program still trying to decide how to measure its intended client outcome (improved fitness); wisely, the staff have chosen not to prematurely set specific targets.

Example 2 shows that one of this facility's objectives was to decrease its annual attrition rate. Over the past year, it had a 38 percent annual attrition rate, which is slightly worse than the industry standard of 35 percent, according to Grantham et al. (1998). Based on member feedback, this program planned to make several changes (e.g., smaller class sizes, staff calls to absent members). The staff hoped these changes would lead to an improvement (decrease) in their member attrition rate of at least 13 percent over the upcoming year.

Examples 4 and 5 both set targets for improving the extent of client benefits (weight loss and rate of reinjury) based on documented outcomes of their programs. Presumably both programs had a justification for expecting that they could improve client outcomes. If nothing changed in the program—either delivery or the type of clientele—one might expect to find similar levels of client outcomes.

A further example of two clinics illustrates that performance targets can be set too low or too high. Programs need to be careful in interpreting performance in terms of success or failure. For instance, Clinic A set out to achieve a 100 percent attendance rate for their rehabilitation program, with the target that 90 percent of their clientele would return to work within three months. They found an 80 percent attendance rate, with 75 percent of clients returning to work. Clinic B set out to achieve a 50 percent attendance rate, with the target that 60 percent of their clientele would return to work within three months. They found 60 percent attendance and 70 percent return to work. Was Clinic A or Clinic B more successful?

A direct comparison suggests that Clinic A produced better rates of participation and results (measured using the indicator return to work). Nonetheless, Clinic A did not meet their performance targets. Clinic B surpassed their targets.

Clearly, it is not productive to speak in terms of program success or failure. Data is value neutral and interpretation of evidence regarding performance accomplishment is always relative: relative to the vested interests of those interpreting the data; relative to the program's objectives; relative to performance targets; relative to past performance; and, in some cases, relative to the performance of other programs. Programs can set targets that may be too high or too low. By documenting performance, programs will be in a position to set more realistic and meaningful performance targets for the upcoming year.

In the example, Clinic A may be satisfied with their program performance and simply wish to maintain the status quo for next year. Clinic B may ask themselves why Clinic A achieved better attendance rates and outcomes. They may find (through process evaluation) that Clinic A offered more flexible scheduling and had a different client profile (for instance, their clientele may be less severely injured). Clinic B may decide to offer more flexible scheduling—something within their control—and strive to improve next year's performance. Although documenting performance accomplishments is the best way to set realistic targets for future performance, programs also need to examine the factors (recruitment, delivery, client characteristics) affecting performance.

Developing a Program Logic Model

A program logic model can also be helpful in evaluation planning. The process of creating a logic model often reveals differences in stakeholder expectations of the program and serves as a starting point for discussion and resolution (Patton 1997; Rossi, Freeman, and Lipsey 1999;

Wholey and Newcomer 1997). A logic model also helps to identify underlying assumptions that you need to examine through evaluation, such as whether providing education results in increased knowledge and, in turn, a change in behavior.

> **A** *logic model* is a diagram illustrating the main components or activities of a program, the objectives and indicators for each activity, and the connections or linkages between them.

Using scenario 5, I have developed a hypothetical program logic model for illustration. Figure 4.2 shows that the primary activities or services provided in this rehabilitation clinic are referral, client assessment, physical conditioning, and client education. Because this program has been operational for some time, it already has most activities in place. However, they are planning to promote the clinic more aggressively to obtain

more physician referrals and develop a back care video to supplement their current education activities (thus, this program has two implementation level objectives).

The output objectives associated with each program activity are expressed as numbers or percentages. Because they have yet to do an evaluation, they have wisely decided not to set arbitrary performance targets. The program decided to consider return to work as an output versus an outcome objective. Note the interrelationship between physical conditioning and back education—both are intended to prevent reoccurrence of injury and chronic (or long-term) back problems. Also, they have separated client outcomes into short-term and long-term objectives. Recall that it is wise to examine short-term or immediate benefits before more long-term outcomes. This simple model can help the rehabilitation clinic determine their priorities for information and focus their evaluation activities accordingly.

Let's say this program is interested in evaluating their education component and decides to do so before putting money into developing and pro-

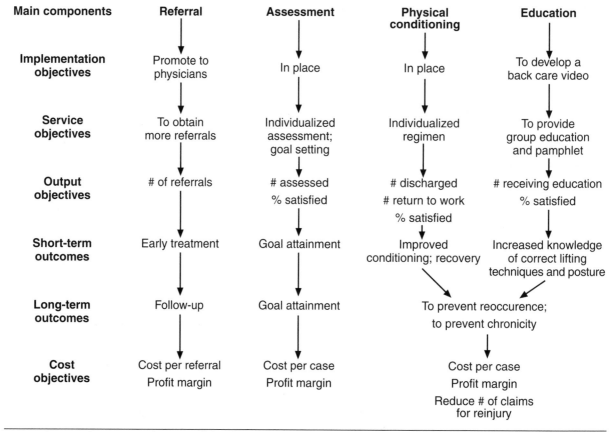

Figure 4.2 Sample program logic model: rehabilitation of injured workers.

ducing a back care video. They may set up a tracking system to record the number of clients who attend the group session and who receive the pamphlet. They may distribute a satisfaction survey, focusing on the education provided. They may hold focus groups with a sample of clients to get in-depth feedback on the perceptions of the group session and pamphlet: Was it understandable? Have they learned anything new? Will they refer to the pamphlet again? They may decide to look for a standardized test to assess knowledge of correct posture and lifting techniques to administer before and after the educational sessions. To examine long-term outcomes, such as reinjury rate, they may decide to follow up with clients by phone a year after they were discharged from the program. As you can see, their logic model served as a useful reference point to guide their evaluation activities. In a multifaceted program with many components and activities, a logic model helps guide evaluation planning.

Summary

This chapter has explained and illustrated each approach to evaluation—needs assessment, formative evaluation, implementation evaluation, process evaluation, outcome evaluation, and cost analysis. Your program's development stage and information needs will dictate which types of evaluation are most relevant and timely.

Carry out your needs assessments during the initial planning stage, but keep in mind that needs assessments are also useful for operational programs to check out the competition and identify possible new markets. I highly recommend formative evaluation, or pilot testing, before full-scale implementation. Implementation evaluation is useful during the start-up phase and simply requires documenting whether and when proposed activities are put into place.

Process and outcome evaluations are vital for programs that are fully operational. Process evaluation examines service delivery and client-usage patterns, and ideally you would conduct it before outcome evaluation so you can make modifications, if necessary and if available resources permit. Outcome evaluation examines the impacts or effects of participation on clients. Programs can do simple types of cost analysis;

however, programs should not consider cost-outcome analysis until they have developed outcome objectives and indicators.

As part of the evaluation planning process, programs also need to examine their aims or objectives—what they want to accomplish. One important task is separating service-oriented and output objectives from client-oriented objectives. Programs need evaluation to document the extent to which they are achieving their various objectives, the most important of which are client outcomes or benefits.

This chapter also examined the process of establishing performance indicators and targets for program objectives. The message is that you should not develop performance targets out of thin air. It is better to have general (and even vague) statements that everyone agrees with, than to set specific performance targets that may look good but have no basis in reality. Documenting your accomplishments regarding service delivery, outputs, and client outcomes through evaluation is the most meaningful way to establish realistic targets for future performance. Finally, a program logic model is a useful tool for describing program activities, for formulating objectives and indicators, and for identifying possible underlying assumptions.

By working through the exercises at the end of this chapter as a team (including representatives of various stakeholder groups whenever possible), you can focus your evaluation activities and prioritize your informational needs. The discussions and debates that will arise may reveal different views, assumptions, and expectations of the program. This is a good thing. By revealing different expectations, you can start to work toward reaching consensus concerning your program objectives and evaluation priorities.

Working Exercises

1. Classify your program or service according to its stage: initial planning, development, early implementation, or fully operational (if so, for how long). Do this exercise, as well as the remaining exercises, separately for each program or service you are involved with.

2. Referring to table 4.1, note the types of evaluation that are best suited to your program's stage and the questions you most want to address.

3. Using worksheet 4.1 describe your program's rationale, list your mission statement or philosophy (if there is one), and start filling in possible objective statements under each category for your program. *Note:* Implementation objectives may not apply at this time if you are not contemplating any new initiatives or activities. Most important, think about what you want your clients to get out of the program (or service), besides being happy campers. How might their lives be different (better, improved) after participating than they were before? What do they tell you is different? How have they changed? Write these in the last box provided in the worksheet. This is the first draft of your client-outcome objective statements.

4. If your program has already developed goal or objective statements, consider whether you have distinct statements concerning client outcomes that are separate from service-oriented objectives and outputs. Have you developed associated indicators and targets? If so, are these targets based on documented past performance, data from other programs, or from the literature?

5. Using worksheet 4.2, start developing your own program logic model. Start by listing each component, activity, or service you provide across the top in a separate column. *Note:* You may have fewer or more activities than the four boxes provided. Next, insert objective statements under each activity. Use arrows to link related activities and related objectives. Beware, however; a logic model is rarely completed in a single attempt. Think of it as a working model that you will refine as your thinking and planning evolve.

6. Prioritize your needs for information: What information do you think is the most important and timely? Who might use such information, besides yourself, and how? What would you like to know first? If others share your priorities, the next order of business is to get the commitment of other stakeholders to the evaluation project you have identified (get them on an evaluation task force).

Worksheet 4.1
Template for Developing Program Objectives

A. Program rationale	**Broad mission statements**
B. Program inputs **B1. Planning**	**Implementation objectives**
B2. Recruitment and delivery	**Process (service) objectives**
C. Program results **C1. Outputs**	**Output objectives**
C2. Outcomes	**Client-oriented (outcome) objectives**

Worksheet 4.2
Template for Developing a Program Logic Model

Main components				
Implementation objectives				
Service objectives				
Output objectives				
Short-term outcomes				
Long-term outcomes				
Cost objectives				

Selecting Your Evaluation Tools

Once you have decided which type of evaluation is the most relevant and timely for your program, the next step is deciding how best to collect the information for your evaluation project.

As you will see, there are many options for data collection. This chapter examines the pros and cons of each option for evaluation purposes. The first section discusses program considerations (issues of feasibility), participant considerations (issues of acceptability and burden), and stakeholder considerations (issues of credibility) in data collection. The second section examines and compares specific data-collection strategies. The final section recommends the most feasible, yet credible, data-collection strategies for programs undertaking their own needs assessment, formative, implementation, process, or outcome evaluations.

Feasibility

Feasibility is a key consideration is selecting your evaluation tools. For instance, programs are unlikely to have the time or expertise necessary to construct and validate their own outcome measures. As you will see, a wide variety of measures are already available for assessing physical and psychological outcomes of exercise for different types of clientele. It is more feasible to select existing outcome tools than to develop your own.

Programs do have to develop, however, their own client-background questionnaires (for process and outcome evaluation) and protocols for surveying potential clients, key informants (for needs assessment), and absent clients or dropouts (as part of process evaluation). Chapter 6

provides templates for background and follow-up questionnaires, protocols for structured telephone surveys, and guidelines for focus groups to help you get started.

Developing data-collection instruments, however, is only one consideration. Personnel time required to administer the instruments (collect the data) is also important in determining which strategies are most feasible for your program. Some data-collection tasks, such as assembling mailing packages, are time consuming but do not require a great deal of training or expertise. You may enlist temporary staff or volunteers for such tasks. This chapter will outline the time, costs, equipment, and expertise required for each data-collection strategy.

Acceptability

You must also consider the demands on the individuals asked to participate in the evaluation—key informants (for needs assessments), potential clients (for needs assessments and formative evaluations), and current and former clients (for process and outcome evaluations). Several factors influence which data-collection strategies are most acceptable from the evaluation participants' perspective.

First, you must give potential participants a good reason for being part of the evaluation. Clients have the right to expect a safe and beneficial program. They also have the right to expect that you will make every attempt to optimize service delivery, such as dealing with overcrowding or scheduling issues. By the same token, they have a responsibility to take part in evaluations aimed at improving program delivery and maximizing benefits. Many clients or potential clients are willing to help programs in their evaluation efforts provided they receive a solid rationale and the program respects their time and confidentiality (Myers 1992).

Tell participants in advance how long the questionnaire, interview, focus group, or fitness assessment is likely to take. As you will see, pilot testing each instrument can help you determine the average time (as well as the maximum and minimum times) required. Participants may want to know the total time commitment required for the entire battery of assessment tools.

You must also weigh each data-collection strategy in terms of client schedules, preferences, and abilities. For instance, busy clients may prefer to fill out a questionnaire at home as opposed to staying after the class to complete the questionnaire on site. Others may prefer a short telephone interview over filling out a questionnaire. People often find it more interesting and less demanding to be part of a focus group discussion rather than an in-depth personal interview, even though both may involve a similar time commitment of one to two hours.

You also need to tailor your data-collection strategies according to the language and literacy, vision and hearing, physical stamina, and cognitive abilities of your clientele. If English is not their first language, you may need to translate questionnaires or enlist interpreters to assist with interviews. Some clients may be comfortable with spoken English but less comfortable reading and writing in English. Such individuals may require assistance with completing questionnaires or scales.

Literacy (reading and writing ability) is an even more sensitive issue. People may be fluent in speaking the language used in the program, but may have difficulty interpreting instructions and items on questionnaires. Given the stigma associated with illiteracy, you must be careful not to embarrass clients when providing assistance for completing questionnaires.

If your clientele is over age 40, remind them to bring their reading glasses if you will give them any type of written questionnaire (including satisfaction surveys). You should also increase the print size, amount of white space (separating questions or sections), and the space provided for open-ended comments on questionnaires. Con-

sider the hearing ability of your clientele when giving verbal instructions for questionnaire completion or when conducting interviews and focus groups.

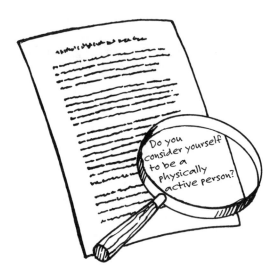

Consider the physical stamina of your clientele. Some clients may have difficulty undergoing demanding physical assessments or sitting for a long time for interviews, focus groups, or questionnaire completion. You may need to shorten assessment protocols or break them into several sessions for such clients. For instance, with some frail clients in the Home Support Exercise Program, we needed to administer a short scale and a mobility test on different days, even though each assessment took only about 15 minutes. When we conducted focus groups with injured workers with low-back pain, we needed to schedule frequent breaks so they could get up and walk around or stretch.

Cognitive abilities are an important consideration when working with clients with dementia or head injuries. Keep self-report measures simple in terms of instructions, rating format, and content. Interview-based administration (versus self-completion) will typically be required. Performance measures with simple instructions are often preferred over self-report measures for such clients (cf. Guralnik et al. 1989).

Credibility

As noted in chapter 4, you may need to justify your evaluation approach to other stakeholders.

You may also need to justify the methods you plan to use to collect the evaluation information.

To enhance the utility of evaluation findings, consult the intended users of the information *before* proceeding with data collection. Obtain input and approval concerning the following:

- The purpose of data collection (type of evaluation and questions to address)
- The rationale for proposed tools and sampling strategies in terms of feasibility, acceptability, and credibility
- The cost and time expected for data collection and analyses
- The type of information that you can obtain from the proposed methods

Justifying evaluation methods and findings after the fact—once you have already collected the data—is risky business. Stakeholders who do not agree with your evaluation findings are likely to attack the credibility of the methods and the resulting information. However, you can enhance the credibility of your findings by using published measures for outcome evaluation, by developing consistent protocols for every type of data collection, by demonstrating sample representativeness, and by explaining unfamiliar data-collection methods to stakeholders during the evaluation project planning stage.

Use Existing Outcome Measures

I strongly recommend using published instruments and assessment protocols for outcome evaluation whenever possible. Such tools have high credibility and may also have accompanying guidelines for administration and scoring. Moreover, using established, published instruments can save you a lot of time; most program leaders or facilities do not have the time or scale-construction expertise to develop their own outcome measures.

To get a measure published, developers must supply evidence to support their tool's reliability and validity; thus, they've already done the work for you. You can reference the published sources in your evaluation proposal (when justifying tool selection) and in your final report (when presenting and interpreting your evaluation findings). I review several published instruments for assessing the physical and psychological benefits of exercise later in this chapter.

Reliability *refers to the consistency or reproducibility of the scores on different testing occasions or by different assessors. Examples of reliability evidence are internal consistency and test-retest reliability (for self-report inventories) and inter-rater and intra-rater reliability (for fitness and performance assessments). Validity addresses the extent to which the measure accurately assesses what it was intended to measure. Examples of validity evidence are comparisons against a recognized, objective standard (criterion validity) or against other existing measures (convergent and discriminant validity). You don't need to understand these technical terms; you just need to cite the references that support the reliability and validity of the measure you intend to use. Face validity—whether the measure looks good for your purposes and is suitable for your clientele—is likely to be your primary selection criteria.*

Consistency in Collection

As noted above, published outcome measures typically have standardized administration guidelines. You need to administer fitness, performance, and self-report measures the same way to all clients, following the scale developer's specific instructions. Likewise, you need to develop a consistent protocol for collecting other types of data.

For instance, the credibility of weight assessment is enhanced if you calibrate the weighing scale and standardize the assessment protocol (e.g., weighing everyone without their shoes) and the recording procedure, such as rounding up scores over .5 to the next highest number.

Chapter 6 shows you how to standardize a background information questionnaire, a protocol for conducting structured telephone interviews, and protocols for conducting focus groups.

Sample Representativeness

Another credibility issue is whether evaluation findings represent the characteristics and perspectives of a program's clientele. Recall that, although you typically give client-satisfaction questionnaires to as many participants as possible, people who have dropped out of the program or are infrequent attenders tend to be under represented in such surveys. As noted in chapter 3, it is important to try and reach these people by surveying at different times (versus only at the last class or session) and mailing the questionnaires to absent members. These strategies can increase your response rate and enhance the representativeness of your survey findings. I present sampling guidelines for various data-collection strategies later in this chapter.

Familiarity With Methods and Information

Stakeholders are more likely to challenge your evaluation findings if they are unfamiliar with the methods you used and the information you're presenting. For instance, you may present quotations from interviews and your audience may ask, "Where are the numbers?" You need to anticipate and address such challenges up front before you collect the data. If you can't convince your stakeholders of the utility of certain types of information in the planning stage, you are unlikely to convince them in the final report.

People tend to be more familiar with, and therefore more comfortable with, numerical, or *quantitative*, data. Everyone has been exposed to gallop polls, market surveys, and election results expressed as numbers, percentages, or rankings. Examples of quantitative information are the number of new or continuing members, the ratio of male to female members, the average age of members, class attendance rates, ratings on client-satisfaction surveys, and scores on fitness assessments or psychological scales.

Examples of *qualitative*, or nonnumerical, data are written responses to open-ended questions and verbal comments made in interviews and focus groups. Some people believe that quantitative information is more objective or less biased than qualitative information. This is simply not true. One is not superior to the other (Mertens 1998; Patton 1997). Qualitative data is more challenging to collect and interpret, but yields rich and detailed information—insights unlikely to emerge from numbers alone.

Similarly, you may view physical data as more objective than information obtained from self-report measures, even though both types of information may be numerical (quantitative).

People trained in exercise physiology and medicine are most familiar with physical indicators such as resting heart rate, blood pressure, or aerobic capacity. Performance measures, such as mobility and balance assessments, familiar to rehabilitation professionals, are now becoming more accepted by nonclinical exercise leaders. In some areas of physical functioning, such as activities of daily living or ADL, there is a choice of performance measures and self-report measures. Direct comparisons of ADL performance and self-reported measures show that one is not superior to the other (cf. Myers et al. 1993).

Furthermore, self-report is the only way to obtain certain types of information, such as self-esteem, body image, perceived well-being, somatic symptoms, pain, and self-efficacy (confidence). As you will see when we review self-report inventories later in this chapter, there are many published (credible) self-report instruments available to evaluate exercise programs.

Despite the tendency to be skeptical of self-report information, the pressure to provide evidence of consumer satisfaction and the widespread use of client-satisfaction surveys has made people familiar with these tools. The advantages of client-satisfaction surveys include

- ease of developing the questionnaire,
- ability to reach a large number of clients,
- a low respondent burden (takes little time to fill out a short satisfaction questionnaire), and
- ease of aggregating and presenting the findings.

Typically, satisfaction results are presented in numerical form (e.g., 85 percent were moderately to highly satisfied with the program). As noted in chapter 3, however, client-satisfaction questionnaires can also include open-ended questions, such as "What do you like most (or least) about the program?" You can present such information as qualitative data (e.g., quotations) or convert it to numerical data (e.g., by counting the number of times clients mentioned specific comments). Having read chapter 3, you realize that client-satisfaction findings are vulnerable to response bias and interpretation problems. This does not mean that programs should not conduct client-satisfaction surveys, but programs need to be aware of, and acknowledge, the limitations of such surveys.

Table 5.1 Features of Various Data-Collection Strategies

Strategy	Client burden	Time and cost	Level of expertise	Reach or # sampled	*Type of evaluation	Type of data
Existing records	None	Low	Low	High	N, I, P, C	Quantitative
Observation: Site visits Case studies	 None High	 Low High	 Low High	 Low Low	 I, P O	Quantitative or qualitative
Questionnaires: On site Mail	 Low Low	 Low Moderate	 Moderate Moderate	 High High	 N, P, O N, P, O	Primarily quantitative
Interviews: Unstructured Structured	 High Low-Mod	 High Moderate	 High Low	 Low Moderate	 N, F, P, O N, F, I, P, O	Primarily qualitative
Focus groups	Moderate	Moderate	Moderate	Moderate	N, F, P	Primarily qualitative
Fitness and performance measures	Mod-High	High	Mod-High	Low-Mod	P, O	Quantitative
Self-report scales	Low-Mod	Low	Low	High	P, O	Quantitative

Note. *Type of evaluation: N = Needs assessment; F = Formative evaluation; I = Implementation evaluation; P = Process evaluation; O = Outcome evaluation; C = Cost analysis.

Credibility issues can arise regardless of whether you collect physical or self-report information or whether you present the data in numerical or nonnumerical form. Once you become familiar with the pros and cons of various information-collection strategies, you will be in a better position to justify your selections to other program stakeholders.

Now that we have examined considerations of feasibility, acceptability, and credibility, let's look at specific data-collection options in more detail. Refer to table 5.1 as we examine each strategy.

Existing Records

As table 5.1 shows, obtaining information from existing records has two attractive features—no client participation is required and program time and cost is minimal, because you have already collected the information. You can use existing records in many types of evaluation. For instance, census lists and public health surveys can provide demographic and health information on your target group for a needs assessment. Directories can help you identify existing exercise services or programs available in your area.

Information for implementation evaluation may be also available from program records. For instance, purchase requisitions and receipts can track equipment costs or repairs, or progress on construction of a new pool. Similarly, it is easy to determine whether new staff have been hired; volunteers trained; or a new pamphlet, poster, or manual developed. For outreach activities, however, site visits are often necessary to determine whether the program has been implemented as originally planned. For instance, in scenario 4 (p. 7), someone from the program should go out and check whether the active living posters were actually put up (and stayed up) in the designated malls.

Some client information for process evaluation may also be available through existing records. You can use routine attendance recording for classes and sign-in logs to calculate participation and adherence rates. You can use information from registration and medical forms to develop client profiles. For instance, in evaluating the Home Support Exercise Program, we obtained information on clients' age, living arrangements, health conditions, use of mobility devices, and medications through case managers (this information was contained in each client's file). Existing records may provide some of, but rarely all, the information you will need for process evaluation. In the above example, we still needed to conduct short interviews with the home care clients because information on exercise habits was not in their files.

For cost analysis, you can break down the total costs of running the program (and time spent with clients) to estimate cost per case. Operating expenses and workload data are often part of routine program record keeping.

Observation

As noted above, observation (through site visits) is a useful strategy for examining whether outreach activities have been implemented. For process evaluation, observing exercise sessions can help you examine class overcrowding and whether clients are correctly performing the exercises or taking their pulses. Periodic observations may be necessary to obtain estimates of member use of exercise equipment and services in large fitness facilities (see chapter 6).

The methodology called *case studies* uses extensive observation and interviewing to describe in detail the effects of an intervention on an individual case (a *case* can be a client or an entire class). This methodology is popular in medicine, counseling, and education. Advanced training is necessary to conduct credible case studies (see Stake 1995 or Yin 1994 for a full description of case study methodology). Few programs have the expertise or time to conduct formal case studies.

It is important not to confuse formal case study evaluation with success stories. Personal testimonials of satisfied clients can be powerful, especially when accompanied by visual images of smiling faces and healthy bodies. Fitness clubs often use before and after pictures in promotional materials showing clients who have dramatically improved their physiques. Rehabilitation programs may describe clients who throw away their walkers. Skeptics are likely to ask, "Are these typical or exceptional cases? How many threw away their walkers? Lost 50 pounds? Were transformed into a Greek god (goddess)?" Success stories provide good illustrations in evaluation reports or presentations. However, you need additional information to convince your audience that these findings are representative. For instance, a more credible success story might read, "Over 75 percent of clients lost at least 25 pounds; one client lost 50 pounds!"

As you will see, functional performance measures, such as balance, are often observation based. Such published performance measures have standardized instructions and rating criteria to guide observers. However, I do not recommend constructing your own observation measures for outcome evaluation for most programs. Credibility of observation information requires evidence of impartiality (objectivity); inter-rater and intra-rater reliability (agreement between different raters observing the same client and agreement between two sets of ratings by the same observer); well-defined rating criteria, such as what constitutes a fall; and verification (e.g., videotapes that others can scrutinize).

Questionnaires

Both program-developed instruments, such as registration forms or client-satisfaction surveys, and published scales (reviewed later in this chapter) come in questionnaire form. Questionnaires with built-in instruction are designed for self-completion. Close-ended questions and forced-choice rating options are preferred over open-ended questions for ease of responding and ease of coding. Thus, information derived from questionnaires tends to be primarily quantitative, or numerical. Questionnaires are a popular and economical strategy for collecting information for needs assessments, process evaluations, and outcome evaluations. Compared with other data-collection strategies, questionnaires are easy to develop, administer, and score and have the highest potential reach (number of people that you can survey). Client burden is generally low, provided the questionnaire is easy and fast to complete.

As table 5.1 shows, you can administer questionnaires on site (at the program) or through the mail. You can do on-site administration individually or in groups. You may simply give clients the questionnaire, ask them to complete it at their convenience (or by a specific date), and return it to the program facility, or you may ask clients to complete questionnaires at the facility during registration or during or after a class session. Group-based administration (usually overseen by one person) tends to enhance the response rate and reduce the amount of missing information. If there is any concern that clients may have difficulty completing questionnaires, having program personnel available for assistance is particularly important. Make sure quiet areas, tables, and pencils are available for on-site completion of questionnaires, and remind clients to bring their reading glasses if needed.

Programs often conduct needs assessment surveys of potential clients through mail or telephone surveys. The biggest challenge is obtaining a list of names and addresses or phone numbers of individuals representative of the intended target group. Random-digit dialing and voter or subscriber lists are often used for general household surveying (by telephone and mail, respectively). Most programs, however, are interested in more specific target audiences, such as certain age groups living in a geographical area. You can use postal codes and area codes to sample a defined region, and you can approach specific groups through schools, work sites, churches, social or recreation centers, shopping malls, or other places where people congregate. The more defined the intended target group (for instance, women working in the textile plant described in scenario 2, p. 7), the easier it is to access a sample.

Mail or telephone surveys are strategies for reaching clients who have left the program or are absent the day of on-site assessment. Usually program mailing and telephone lists already exist for reaching current or previous clients. Update client mailing and telephone lists every few months because people may move.

Take into account costs for envelopes, postage, and personnel time to assemble packages when mailing questionnaires. Computer-generated mailing labels save time. Generally, the response rate for mailed questionnaires tends to be lower than those administered on site. Strategies for increasing the return rate for mailed questionnaires include

- enclosing a personalized cover letter,
- including a stamped return envelope,
- sending out a reminder postcard about a week after the first mailing, and
- sending out further packages by registered mail.

Increasing the response rate of telephone surveys involves repeated callbacks at different times of the day and evening and on different days of the week. (See Dillman 1978, an excellent resource for mail and telephone surveys.)

> **S**urveying by e-mail is becoming an increasingly popular, low-cost alternative to mail and fax surveys. Similar to mail surveys, however, e-mail surveys require lists, and you must personalize your survey. Most of us discard junk e-mail as quickly as junk snail mail without even opening the message.

Interviews

Questionnaires tend to be highly structured. Interviews, meanwhile, can be highly structured, semistructured, or unstructured. The more unstructured the interview, the greater the expertise required (cf. Kvale 1996; Mertens 1998). When used as the primary data-collection strategy, personal interviews tend to be unstructured and intensive, often lasting several hours and repeated on several occasions. Interpreting the complex qualitative information from multiple, individual interviews requires special training and experience (Kvale 1996). In-depth, one-on-one interviews are demanding for the interviewer and the interviewee.

For the reasons above, classic interviewing is not feasible for most programs as a primary evaluation tool. However, you can use highly structured interviews in place of questionnaires in several situations. As mentioned, clients unable to complete a questionnaire on their own (due to language, literacy, or vision problems) may need assistance. The structured questionnaire is still the data-collection instrument; you are simply administering the tool by reading the instructions, items, and response options out loud to assist clients.

Highly structured interviews conducted by telephone are more similar to questionnaires than to classic interviewing. The surveyor or interviewer reads the questions over the phone and records the responses. Keep the list of rating options short and simple for telephone surveys. Telephone surveys can be an efficient alternative to mail surveys when obtaining information for needs assessment (from key informants and potential clients) and for process evaluation (from absent members). Chapter 6 contains a short and easy telephone protocol for contacting and assessing absent members.

Focus Groups

Although sometimes called group interviews, focus groups differ from classic interviews in several respects. First, focus groups tend to be more structured than interviews. Second, each person is only asked to take part in one focus group discussion session, as opposed to the multiple sessions required for classic interviews. Third, focus groups involve interaction and exchange of ideas *among* participants (in contrast to the limited two-way interaction in individual interviews). The dynamic nature of focus group discussions encourages differences of opinion on the topics or issues and provides the opportunity for participants to reconsider their initial opinions or impressions in light of comments made by other participants (Krueger 1994; Mertens 1998).

Focus groups can be especially useful when you want to obtain the reactions of *potential clients* to a new program (needs assessment) or to draft program materials (formative evaluation), or when you want detailed feedback from *current clients* on perceived barriers to participation or their suggestions on expanding or reducing services (process evaluation).

Compared with other data-collection strategies, focus groups are rated as moderate with respect to client burden, time and cost, level of expertise

required, and reach (see table 5.1). Because focus groups typically include 6 to 12 people per session, it is a more economical strategy than individual interviewing. Focus groups can also seem less demanding to participants in that each participant decides when and how much he or she wishes to contribute to the discussion. Because focus groups are the best strategy for obtaining detailed client feedback for needs assessments, and formative and process evaluations, chapter 6 provides you with explicit, step-by-step guidelines for conducting focus groups.

Fitness and Performance Measures

A wide variety of credible, published tools are available for assessing the physical and psychological outcomes of exercise. Your task is to select those that best address your program's intended outcomes, are suitable for your clientele, and are feasible to administer. This section describes some fitness and functional performance measures available for measuring the physical benefits of exercise. The next section describes some self-report scales that measure physical activity, psychological outcomes such as self-confidence, functional ability or disability, health status, and well-being.

Fitness Assessments

Many programs provide *fitness appraisals* or *fitness assessments*—a battery of fitness measures that evaluate cardiorespiratory endurance, muscular strength and endurance, flexibility, and body composition—as a client service. Programs often use initial assessments for screening and developing individualized exercise prescriptions. You can use reappraisals, when conducted, to provide personalized feedback on client progress. In programs with an aerobic component, instructors often teach clients how to take their pulses and use charts on target heart rates and perceived exertion. Van Norman (1995) recommends that fitness program leaders record exercise and recovery heart rates for every student over the first few weeks for safety and to reinforce participant self-monitoring.

You can also use information from fitness assessments for process evaluation (to profile your clientele according to initial fitness levels). If you conduct fitness assessments consistently across clients, and periodically reassess clients, such information may also be useful for outcome evaluation. For instance, comparing pre- and postexercise resting heart rate is a simple and quick indicator of improved fitness. Recommended fitness assessment protocols vary depending on whether you refer to guidelines published by the American College of Sports Medicine (ACSM), the Canadian Society for Exercise Physiology (CSEP), the American Council on Exercise (ACE), or guidelines of other associations. Equipment requirements also vary by protocol. For instance, you can assess body composition using a weight scale and tape measure, skin fold calipers, or underwater weighing tanks.

Some groups provide reference or normative data to assist with interpreting client scores. For instance, the Canadian Physical Activity, Fitness and Life-style appraisal battery provides normative anthropometric and performance data for apparently healthy men and women aged 15 to 69 (CSEP 1996). The National Health and Nutrition Examination Surveys (Frisancho 1990) in the United States provide anthropometric reference data for Hispanic, white, and African American populations.

Maximal oxygen uptake, or $\dot{V}O_2$max, is considered the gold standard, or the most accurate and reliable measure of physical fitness with respect to cardiorespiratory or aerobic capacity. Most nonclinical fitness programs do not have the equipment or medical personnel recommended (e.g., by ACSM 1997a) for such testing. Submaximal aerobic testing (shown to correlate with $\dot{V}O_2$max), however, is feasible for most programs. Such testing can range from protocols using a stationary bicycle or treadmill to even simpler step or walking protocols. When conducting fitness assessments, consider whether you have the training or expertise, as well as the equipment and space required. Keep in mind that the fitness assessment protocol should be standardized or consistent across clients and that you should regularly check and calibrate equipment.

As in scenario 9 (p. 9), the personal trainer starting his own business has decided to target persons aged 40 to 69. He advertises the following services: fitness appraisals, supervised exercise sessions, massage therapy, and weight and stress management. Having been trained as a Certified Fitness Consultant by the CSEP, he is familiar with their battery of tests and norms for healthy adults aged 15 to 69 (CSEP 1996). He intends to work out of his mobile van. So, due to space limitations, he decides to use a step test protocol for assessing submaximal aerobic fitness. He will hold off on purchasing more expensive skin fold calipers for now. From height and weight he can calculate body mass index. Waist girth provides an indicator of trunk adiposity (and is a recognized risk factor for heart disease). If individual clients are particularly interested in losing inches from their hips or thighs, or increasing their biceps through weight training, he takes additional girth measurements for those clients. For musculoskeletal fitness, he plans to follow CSEP's push-up and curl-up protocols (except for clients with back pain). For flexibility, he'll use the sit-and-reach test. The CSEP guide does not cover stress measurement, so he decides to search the Internet for possible measures related to stress reduction or relaxation. Because building his client base depends largely on physician referral, he reconsiders his tool kit in terms of what physicians might like to know. Because he thinks physicians will be interested in such results, he decides to add resting heart rate and blood pressure to his tool kit. This personal trainer has made careful, pragmatic decisions in selecting his assessment battery. He has considered the informational needs of three stakeholder groups:

1. What his clients want to know (their individual progress)
2. What he needs to know (for screening and evaluation)
3. What physicians want to know (when judging the merit of his services)

In addition to feasibility, consider the suitability of fitness assessments for your clientele. If you work with older adults (other than masters athletes), traditional ways of assessing cardiorespiratory fitness, such as treadmill or cycle endurance tests, or muscular strength, using one-repetition maximum (1-RM) strength tests, are unsuitable (Rikkli and Jones 1997; Spirduso 1995). In the over age 75 category, it is estimated that only 5 percent are in the physically fit and elite category (Spirduso 1995). Unfit, middle-aged adults, particularly those with chronic health conditions, such as heart disease or diabetes, may similarly be unable or unwilling to undergo fitness tests designed for younger adults. Measures of endurance, strength, and flexibility have been developed specifically for unfit middle-aged and older adults. For instance, a modified sit-and-reach test that clients can do in a chair or wheelchair is available to assess flexibility in persons unable to get on the floor (Lazowski et al. 1997). As described in the next section, measures of functional performance are commonly used with older clientele.

Functional Performance Measures

In the exercise field, performance refers to *task performance,* such as number of sit-ups or curl-ups, and *athletic performance,* such as running times, swimming times, or skills. *Functional performance,* also called functional fitness, refers specifically to "the ability to respond to the physical demands of daily living with vigor and without undue fatigue, and still have enough reserve energy to engage in leisurely pursuits" (Caspersen, Powell, and Christensen 1985).

To live independently, one must be able to carry groceries, safely cross an intersection, avoid a fall, and so on. Preventing illness and accidents and maintaining physical abilities despite common, chronic conditions, such as arthritis, are important to most older adults (World Health Organization [WHO] 1997). Functional ability as opposed to physical fitness is the primary objective of many exercise and rehabilitation programs for middle-aged and older adults.

An array of published functional performance measures are available, including tests of endurance, strength, flexibility, mobility (locomotion, balance, gait), reaction times, manual abilities, and self-care abilities. Many tests have been developed in the rehabilitation field by physical and occupational therapists. The Canadian Physiotherapy Association (1994) has published a manual containing over 50 functional performance and self-report measures for various client groups. Spirduso's (1995) book contains an excellent review of performance tests for older adults along the continuum of fitness and frailty. Table 5.2 presents examples of validated, published functional performance measures that have been used as outcome measures in exercise interventions.

As you can see in the right column of table 5.2, some functional performance measures are

suitable for higher functioning older adults and others are more suitable for frail or lower functioning older adults. Some measures in the former category, such as the half-mile timed walk test in the Osness et al. (1990) battery, are also suitable for unfit middle-aged adults.

Self-Report Scales

I've noted that performance measures are not superior to self-report measures. Further, some information, such as physical activity patterns and psychological well-being, can only be obtained using self-report measures. Table 5.3 lists several types of published self-report scales applicable for measuring potential outcomes of exercise programs.

Physical Activity Questionnaires

For both marketing and evaluation purposes, it is useful to know how physically active your clientele are when they enter your program. Are you attracting active individuals, sedentary individuals, or a mixture of both? You can measure physical fitness and infer that more fit individuals are already physically active. However, genetic makeup and other life-style practices, such as smoking and diet, also play a role in fitness level. Information on health behaviors is usually obtained through self-report. Although it is simple to inquire about smoking status, determining patterns of physical activity is complex, as you will see.

A collection of 28 published physical activity questionnaires is contained in the June 1997 supplement of *Medicine & Science in Sports & Exercise* (Kriska and Caspersen 1997). The publication presents each instrument in its entirety, reviews evidence for validity and reliability, and provides instructions for administration and scoring.

Unfortunately, most physical activity questionnaires have been developed for research purposes and are time consuming to complete (client burden) and code (administration burden). Table 5.3 references a few measures contained in the supplement. The Bouchard Three-Day Record, for instance, requires an individual to record for each 15-minute period (over a 24-hour cycle for each of three consecutive days) the type of activity engaged in (e.g., lying down to sleep; stand-

Table 5.2 Sample Functional Performance Measures

Measure	Source	Focus	Suitability
AAHPERD Functional Fitness Assessment Battery	Osness et al. (1990)	Aerobic endurance, muscle strength and endurance, flexibility, coordination, and agility	Adults 60+, higher functioning
SpeciFit Walk Test and Strength	Cotton, Ekeroth, and Yancy (1998) ACE Guide	Endurance, strength, and range of motion	Older adults, moderate to high functioning
Paced Walk Test	Himman et al. (1988)	Slow, normal, and fast gait speed	Adults 55+, moderate to high functioning
Timed Up-and-Go (TUG) Test	Podsiadlo and Richardson (1991)	Mobility	Adults 70+, lower functioning
Berg Balance Scale	Berg et al. (1989)	Balance	Moderate to lower functioning
Tinetti Balance and Gait Assessment	Tinetti (1986)	Balance and gait	Moderate to lower functioning
Sit to Stands Walking/Wheelchair Propulsion	Schnelle et al. (1995)	Mobility and endurance	Low functioning
Functional Independence Measure (FIM)	Granger and Hamilton (1993)	Self-care, transfers, locomotion, memory, communication	Low functioning
Modified Sit and Reach	Lazowski et al. (1997)	Flexibility	Persons with difficulty on traditional test
Belt-Resisted Strength Measures	Desrosiers et al. (1998)	Upper and lower extremity strength	Range of functioning
Functional Reach	Duncan et al. (1990)	Stability and reach	Range of functioning

ing doing light, moderate, and intense activities, for example, manual work, sports, and leisure). The person's body weight is used to estimate daily energy expenditure (in kilocalories). The Modified Activity Questionnaire (MAQ) asks respondents to recall the number of times per month over the past year (and average minutes per time) that they jogged, swam, and so on (from a list of 40 activities). Total activity, leisure activity, and occupational activity scores on the MAQ are expressed in METs (metabolic equivalents).

Descriptions of these two measures show you how complex it is to accurately estimate physical activity patterns, taking into account work and leisure, as well as frequency, intensity, and duration of the activities. There are simpler assessments, such as the three questions contained in CSEP's (1996) Healthy Physical Activity Participation Questionnaire:

1. Over a typical seven-day period, how many times do you engage in physical activity that is

Table 5.3 Self-Report Scales Applicable to Exercise

Category	Measure	Source	Number of items
Physical activity	Bouchard Three-Day Record	Bouchard et al. (1983)	8 activity codes, 15 min recording
	Modifiable Activity Questionnaire (MAQ)	Kriska and Bennett (1992)	7 items (5 categorical, 2 require listings)
	Physical Activity Scale for the Elderly (PASE)	Washburn et al. (1993)	10 items
	Older Adult-Exercise Status Inventory (OA-ESI)	O'Brien Cousins (1997)	44 items
	Healthy Physical Activity Participation Questionnaire	Canadian Society of Exercise Physiology (CSEP 1996)	3 items
Self-efficacy	Physical Activity Efficacy Scale	McAuley, Lox, and Duncan (1993)	27 items
	Adherence Efficacy Scale	McAuley, Lox, and Duncan (1993)	12 items
	Barriers to Exercise Scale	McAuley and Jacobson (1991)	13 items
	Self-Efficacy for Cardiac Patients	Ewart et al. (1986)	6 items
	Self-Efficacy for COPD Patients	Kaplan, Atkins, and Reinsch (1984)	7 items
	Diabetes Self-Efficacy Scale (DSES)	Padgett (1991)	19 items
	Functional Abilities Confidence Scale (FACS) for injured workers	Williams and Myers (1998b)	15 items
	Arthritis Self-Efficacy Scale	Lorig et al. (1989)	20 items
	Falls Efficacy Scale (FES)	Tinetti, Richman, and Powell (1990)	10 items

	Activities-Specific Balance Confidence (ABC) Scale	Powell and Myers (1995); Myers et al. (1996, 1998)	16 items
Functional ability/disability	Arthitic Impact Measurement Scale (AIMS)	Meenan (1982)	45 items
	Osteoporosis Functional Disability Questionnaire (OFDQ)	Helmes et al. (1995)	71 items
	Roland-Morris Disability Questionnaire	Roland and Morris (1983)	24 items
	Resumption of Activities of Daily Living (RADL) Scale	Williams and Myers (1998a)	12 items
Health-status and well-being	Subjective Exercise Experiences Scale (SEES)	McAuley and Courneya (1994)	12 items
	Exercise-Induced Feeling Inventory (EFI)	Gauvin and Rejeski (1993)	12 items
	Pittsburg Sleep Quality Index (PSEQ)	Buysse et al. (1989)	19 items
	SF-36 Health Survey	McHorney, Ware, and Raczek (1993)	36 items
	Vitality Plus Scale (VPS)	Myers et al. (in press)	10 items

sufficiently prolonged and intense to cause sweating and a rapid heart beat? (at least three times, normally once or twice, rarely or never).

2. When you engage in physical activity, do you have the impression that you make an intense effort, make a moderate effort, or make a light effort?

3. In a general fashion, would you say that your current physical fitness is very good, good, average, poor, very poor?

Frequency, intensity, and perceived fitness are scored and summarized into a health benefit zone ranging from excellent to needs improvement.

This questionnaire has not been validated, however, and is intended as a client screening and motivational tool rather than as a tool for assessing change (CSEP 1996).

Self-Efficacy Measures

Self-efficacy (or confidence) is a key factor concerning exercise adherence. Self-efficacy for exercise predicts adherence (i.e., less confident individuals are more likely to discontinue the exercise regimen). Self-efficacy can be enhanced by exercise participation; thus, you can also use

Figure 5.1
The Activities-Specific Balance Confidence (ABC) Scale

For *each* of the following activities, please indicate your level of self-confidence by choosing a corresponding number from the following rating scale:

0%   10   20   30   40   50   60   70   80   90   100%
No confidence   Completely confident

How confident are you that you can maintain your balance and remain steady when you . . .

1. walk around the house? _____ %

2. walk up or down stairs? _____%

3. bend over and pick up a slipper from the front of a closet floor? _____%

4. reach for a small can off a shelf at eye level? _____%

5. stand on your tip toes and reach for something above your head? _____%

6. stand on a chair and reach for something? _____%

7. sweep the floor? _____%

8. walk outside the house to a car parked in the driveway? _____%

9. get into or out of a car? _____%

10. walk across a parking lot to the mall? _____%

11. walk up or down a ramp? _____%

12. walk in a crowded mall where people rapidly walk past you? _____%

13. are bumped into by people as you walk through the mall? _____%

14. step on or off an escalator while holding onto a railing? _____%

15. step on or off an escalator while holding parcels and cannot hold onto the railing? _____%

16. walk outside on icy sidewalks? _____%

Note. From Powell and Myers (1995), Myers et al. (1996), and Myers et al. (1998). Reprinted with permission of the Gerontology Society of America. Copyright by the GSA.

Administrating the ABC

The ABC can be self-administered or administered via personal or telephone interview. Use a larger typeset font for self-administration, while an enlarged version of the rating scale on an index card will facilitate in-person interviews. Instruct respondents, "If you **do not currently do** the activity in question, try to imagine how confident you would be if you had to do the activity. If you normally use a walking aid or hold onto someone, rate your confidence as if you were using these supports. If you have any questions, please ask."

Instructions for Scoring

Total the ratings (possible range = 0 to 1,600) and divide by 16 (or the number of items completed) to get each person's ABC score. If a person qualifies her response to items 2, 9, 11, 14, or 15, solicit separate ratings and use the *lowest* confidence of the two (as this will limit the entire activity, e.g., likelihood of using stairs). Total scores can be computed if at least 12 of the 16 items are answered and alpha does not decrease appreciably with the deletion of item 16— icy sidewalks—for administration in warmer climates (Myers et al. 1998).

Psychometric Properties of the ABC Scale

The ABC has good test-retest reliability, high internal consistency, is able to discriminate between fallers and nonfallers and low versus high mobility groups (Powell and Myers 1995), and corresponds with balance performance measures (Myers et al. 1996). ABC scores above 50 and less than 80 are indicative of a moderate level of functioning characteristic of persons with chronic health conditions. Scores above 80 indicate higher functioning, usually active older adults and are achievable through exercise and rehabilitative therapies (Myers et al. 1998).

self-efficacy as an outcome measure. As table 5.3 shows, there are several self-efficacy measures developed for different purposes and populations.

The Physical Activity Efficacy Scale asks respondents to rate their level of self-confidence regarding various distances they can walk or jog in a specified time, the number of sit-ups they can do (from 1 to 50), and how long they can ride a stationary bike without discomfort or stopping. The Adherence Efficacy Scale assesses whether people feel confident they can continue to exercise for 40+ minutes, three times a week at moderate intensity for the next two weeks, next four weeks, and so on up to six months.

The Barriers to Exercise Scale assesses whether persons feel confident (from 0 percent = not at all confident to 100 percent = completely confident) they can continue to exercise three times per week under different conditions—bad weather, bored with the program or activity, on vacation, exercising alone, feeling self-conscious, if it became difficult to get to the location, if the instructor did not offer any encouragement, and so on. All three scales have been used with young to middle-aged adults to predict exercise adherence.

Keep in mind, however, that self-efficacy is situation specific, and you must tailor it to the exercise regimen and clientele in question. For instance, Ewart et al. (1986) and Kaplan, Atkins, and Reinsch (1984) developed self-efficacy measures based on exercise regimens tailored for persons with heart disease and chronic obstructive pulmonary diseases (COPD), respectively.

Other self-efficacy measures focus on multiple components of disease self-management. For instance, the Diabetes Self-Efficacy Scale (DSES) examines confidence concerning exercise, diet, glucose monitoring, and so on. Still other self-efficacy measures do not focus on exercise per se (e.g., the Arthritis Self-Efficacy Scale

and the Functional Abilities Confidence Scale [FACS] for injured workers), but have been used as outcome measures in exercise interventions.

Because falling is a concern of many older adults, and exercise may improve balance ability and confidence, programs for older adults should consider using balance performance and self-efficacy measures. The Falls Efficacy Scale (FES) focuses on simple daily-living situations, such as taking a bath or shower and getting dressed, and is an appropriate measure for lower functioning seniors. The Activities-Specific Balance Confidence (ABC) Scale, in contrast, was developed for higher functioning seniors and includes more challenging daily living situations. Figure 5.1 shows the ABC scale to illustrate a self-efficacy scale.

The 0 percent (no confidence) to 100 percent (complete confidence) rating format for the ABC scale is typical of most self-efficacy measures. The ABC has been used in several evaluations of community and rehabilitation exercise programs for older adults (Myers et al. 1998). The ABC is an appropriate tool to consider for scenarios 3 (Tai Chi), 4 (mall-walking program), and 8 (wellness clinics).

Functional Ability or Disability

Many exercise and rehabilitation programs, particularly those for seniors and persons with injuries or chronic conditions, state that their primary objective is to restore or maintain the level of client functioning. There is an array of published self-report measures to assess functional ability (disability) or limitations in activities of daily living. Some examples for specific populations are shown in table 5.3. For instance, the Roland-Morris and the Resumption of Activities of Daily Living (RADL) scales were developed for use with rehabilitation clients with low-back pain (LBP).

One difficulty with performance and self-report measures of functioning is they do not capture a person's level of functioning before the injury, accident, stroke, and so on. A focus group of injured workers with LBP told us that for them, "Recovery means getting back to the way I was before the injury" or "getting back to normal." Accordingly, we developed the RADL Scale to assess the extent to which injured workers resumed their usual activities in several domains (sleeping, sexual activity, chores, work, etc.). This scale allows clinicians to determine how much recovery has taken place between the time of injury and entry into the rehabilitation program. We found that both physical conditioning and RADL scores improved over three weeks in an exercise and education rehabilitation program for many clients (Williams and Myers 1998a). The RADL would be a good tool for scenario 5 (the rehabilitation clinic under accreditation).

Figure 5.2
Vitality Plus Scale (VPS)

This scale looks at how you are **currently feeling**. For each statement, circle a number from 1 to 5 that best describes you. For instance, if you usually fall asleep quickly then you want to circle 5. Otherwise, circle a number from 1 to 4, depending on the extent to which you usually have difficulty falling asleep.

	1	2	3	4	5	
Take a long time to fall asleep	1	2	3	4	5	Fall asleep quickly
Sleep poorly	1	2	3	4	5	Sleep well
Tired or drowsy during the day	1	2	3	4	5	Feel rested
Rarely hungry	1	2	3	4	5	Excellent appetite
Often constipated	1	2	3	4	5	Do not get constipated
Often have aches & pains	1	2	3	4	5	Have no aches & pains
Low energy level	1	2	3	4	5	Full of pep and energy
Often stiff in the morning	1	2	3	4	5	Not stiff in the morning
Often restless or agitated	1	2	3	4	5	Feel relaxed
Often do not feel good	1	2	3	4	5	Feel good

Note. From "Measuring accumulated health-related benefits of exercise participation by older adults: The Vitality Plus Scale" by A.M. Myers et al., in press. Reprinted by permission of the Gerontological Society of America. Copyright by the GSA.

Administering the Vitality Plus Scale (VPS)

The VPS can be self-administered or administered via personal or telephone interview. Use larger size fonts if you are gathering the responses from older persons, and use an enlarged rating scale on an index card to facilitate interview-assisted administration. Query each respondent to ensure they understand the instructions and rating format.

Instructions for Scoring the VPS

Each item is scored from 1 to 5 based on the respondent's rating. Calculate a total Vitality Plus Score by summarizing the item scores. Total scores can range from 10 to 50 with higher scores indicating greater well-being. Do not compute total scores unless an individual has answered at least 7 items. Substitute the mean (total divided by number of items answered) for the missing values to compute a total score.

Psychometric Properties of the Vitality Plus Scale

The VPS was developed and validated using exercise and nonexercise groups composed of both middle-age and older adults (Myers et al. in press). The scale has good internal consistency and test-retest reliability. Scale scores are correlated with gait speed and mobility, related to subscales of the SF-36, and responsive to change for individuals with low to moderate scores prior to participation in a variety of exercise programs (including aerobics classes, strength training, Tai Chi, aquatics, and walking). Improvement is more likely for individuals who are older, more sedentary, and have health problems since these individuals are likely to score lower at baseline and have more room for improvement (Myers et al. in press).

Health Status and Well-Being

Recall that according to surveys, the primary reasons people say they exercise is to look and feel better. Functional ability measures focus on pain, mobility, and other limitations in performing daily activities. Certainly, exercise can improve physical condition and reduce the limitations associated with low-back pain, arthritis, osteoporosis, and other health conditions. Exercise can also help people sleep better, feel more relaxed, increase energy levels, and enhance overall quality of life or well-being (Rejeski, Brawley, and Shumaker 1996).

As table 5.3 shows, two short measures—the Subjective Exercise Experiences Scale (SEES) and the Exercise-Induced Feeling Inventory (EFI)—assess whether participants feel fatigued, worn out, crummy, discouraged or energetic, refreshed, calm, relaxed, positive, or terrific immediately following a bout of exercise. Such scales may be useful to identify early dropouts; however, regular exercisers tend to report high scores for the positive items and low scores for the negative items.

Many general measures of psychological well-being are available (cf. McDowell and Newell 1996) and have been used in exercise research studies to evaluate outcomes of exercise programs. In fact, a review by McAuley and Rudolph (1995) found that over 85 different psychological scales have been used in published exercise studies. The general consensus is that measures of life satisfaction or self-esteem are too global as exercise outcomes, and measures of anxiety or depression are not appropriate for psychologically healthy adults (McAuley and Rudolph 1995; Myers et al. in press; Rejeski, Brawley, and Shumaker 1996; Stewart and King 1991).

Table 5.4 Recommended Data-Collection Strategies and Sampling Guidelines

Type of evaluation Source of information	Data-collection strategies	Sampling guidelines
Needs assessments		
Demographic indicators	Existing survey data	All available
Existing services	Directories, yellow pages	All available
Key informants	Structured survey or interview	All or representative sample
Potential clients	Mail or phone survey	100 surveys
	Focus groups	2 to 6 groups
Formative evaluation		
Potential clients	Focus groups	2 to 6 groups
Implementation evaluation		
Planned on-site activities	Program records, minutes	All relevant
	Observation	Random selection
	Staff interviews	All involved
Planned outreach activities	Site visits	All outreach activities
Process evaluation		
Client profile	Background questionnaire	All clients
Participation rates	Attendance records or logs	All clients
Client feedback	Satisfaction questionnaire	All clients
	Focus groups	2 to 6 groups
Dropout characteristics	Background questionnaire	All clients
Dropout feedback	Structured telephone protocol	As many as possible
Outcome evaluation		
Selecting measures	Pilot testing	5 to 10 clients
Pre- and postassessment	Published inventories and fitness/performance measures	At least 30 clients

There are existing measures that focus on specific parameters of well-being such as sleep quality. Studies have shown that regular exercisers report less sleep disturbance and that participation in a moderate intensity exercise program can lead to sleep improvement in about 16 weeks (Brassington and Hicks 1995; King et al. 1997). There are also more extensive measures, such as the SF-36 Health Survey (McHorney 1996), which assess physical, social, and emotional functioning. A more user-friendly measure, the Vitality Plus Scale (VPS, figure 5.2) is now available to measure various components of feeling good in a single, short measure developed specifically for exercise programs with middle-aged and older adults. In chapter 7, I'll use the VPS to show you how to code and analyze data from self-report scales.

Pilot Testing

Regardless of which measures you choose for your outcome evaluation, you must first pilot test the measure with your clientele. Pilot testing requires only a small number of clients (5 to 10). For your pilot group, choose some of your highest functioning and some of your lowest functioning clients to see whether there are floor or ceiling effects. A *floor effect* occurs when the measure is too difficult and some clients cannot complete the assessment (and receive a score). For instance, Rikkli and Jones (1997) expressed this concern with the half-mile walk test—some older adults cannot walk this distance. Conversely, a *ceiling effect* occurs when the test is too easy and many clients receive perfect or top scores. For instance, look at the ABC scale in figure 5.1. If your pilot group all score high (90 percent to 100 percent), indicating complete confidence in these activities, the ABC scale is too easy for them. Conversely, if all your clients score low (0 percent or no confidence) and remark that they do not do these activities any more, you should consider another measure, such as, in this case, the FES. An outcome measure also should be able to distinguish between clients. Score the measure for your pilot sample and see whether you get a range of scores. Clarity of instructions and time taken to administer and complete each tool should also be determined through pilot testing.

Pilot testing is also recommended for all newly developed mail and telephone surveys and client-background and satisfaction questionnaires. The purpose here is to make sure that the instructions and items are clear and easy to interpret. For your pilot sample, record the time for individuals to complete each tool to determine the minimum, maximum (range), and average. Tell your pilot group how you intend to use the measure and get their input on the suitability and relevance of the measure. Be sensitive to language, literacy, and visual abilities as well as the other client factors that may influence willingness and ability to complete your evaluation tools.

Recommended Strategies for Evaluation

This chapter presents a great deal of information concerning various options for data collection. To help you digest all this information, table 5.4 summarizes the data-collection strategies recommended throughout this chapter for specific types of evaluation.

My recommendations assume that most of you will be conducting your own evaluations. Therefore, you need to use the most practical data-collection strategies. Table 5.4 also contains sampling guidelines explained below as we review each type of evaluation.

For needs assessments, access all available demographic information on your target group and on existing services in your area. There may be only a small number of key informants in your community who have expertise concerning the type of service or program you are considering offering. If so, survey as many key informants as possible. One key informant will refer you to another (the snowball sampling technique). Decide on a few important questions you want to ask your key informants:

- What types of services do they provide?
- What is the nature and the size of their client base?
- What are their recruitment strategies?

Then, set up times to meet or talk with these individuals and use your list of questions to guide your structured interviews in person or over the phone.

To obtain the input of potential clients, you have three options: mail surveys, structured telephone surveys (based on simple questionnaire protocols), or focus groups. It is easier to reach respondents through mailed surveys than through phone surveys (because more personnel time is required for the latter). A sample size of about 100 is required for a general mail or phone survey (Mertens 1998). Make sure that the sample is representative. For instance, if you want to attract both men and women to your program, make sure that you include both groups in your survey.

A significantly smaller sample size is one reason focus groups are so appealing. Six to 12 people participate in each focus group (at one time). Most experts recommend that you conduct at least two focus groups for an evaluation project (Krueger 1994; Mertens 1998; Morgan 1993), but you may require up to six (see chapter 6).

Provided you can get potential clients to come to a central location to participate, focus groups are a preferred strategy over mail or telephone surveys for obtaining the input of potential clients for needs assessment and formative evaluation, and for obtaining the feedback of current clients for process evaluations.

For implementation evaluation, you can use records, such as purchase invoices, along with observation of on-site projects, such as a swimming pool under construction, and visits to off-site projects.

Remember to also obtain a profile of all clients in your program, including background characteristics and attendance, participation, or usage rates. You can obtain client feedback through satisfaction surveys and focus groups. You can also examine the characteristics of continuing members versus dropouts if all clients complete a background questionnaire when they enter the program. I recommend a structured telephone survey to determine reasons for absence or dropout (see chapter 6).

Use existing, published fitness, performance, and self-report scales for outcome evaluation. Pilot-test potential measures before starting the outcome study. Then, administer each measure at least twice, at baseline or program entry and after some period of participation, to determine change. I further discuss sample selection, timing of assessments, and calculating change in chapters 6 and 7.

Summary

Clearly, there are several trade-offs in choosing one data-collection strategy over another. However, now that you are aware of the pros and cons of each strategy, you are better able to select tools that are feasible for your evaluation projects and acceptable to your clientele. You should also be better prepared to justify your selection of data-collection methods to other stakeholders if

necessary. You may still be unfamiliar with the focus group strategy. Chapter 6 provides a thorough description of what is involved and the richness of the information that you can obtain through focus groups.

For outcome evaluation, use published tools and assessment protocols whenever possible. This chapter described an array of fitness assessment protocols, performance measures, and self-report inventories applicable to the exercise field. The tools provide a solid starting point for most exercise programs. Once you find an outcome evaluation tool that meets your needs, you probably will stick with it for some time, but keep in mind that new measures for various populations are always emerging in the exercise and rehabilitation fields.

You can go to a university or hospital library or use on-line search engines available on the Internet to find published measures. Medline (**http://www.nlm.nih.gov/databases/medline.html**) is a good database to search for measures appropriate to the exercise field. Key word searches by topic (e.g., strength measures) and client characteristics, such as older adults, diabetics, osteoporosis, and cardiac rehabilitation, will produce lists of sources and an abstract for each article.

Being able to cite published references regarding the established validity and reliability for your outcome tools (in your evaluation proposal and the final report) will add scientific credibility to your tool selection. You do not need to understand the technical terms. Face validity, or whether the measure looks good for your purposes, is likely to be your primary selection criteria. Remember to always pilot test the proposed tool with your clientele to determine perceived relevance, clarity, ease of completion (and administration), and to see whether the measure is too hard or too easy for your clientele (floor and ceiling effects).

Working Exercises

1. Take an inventory of the fitness assessment protocols, medical forms, registration forms, client-satisfaction surveys, and any other tools you currently use to collect client information.

2. Take an inventory of your program or facility's available fitness assessment equipment. Take an inventory of your personnel. Who is currently responsible for administering fitness assessments, medical histories, client-satisfaction forms, and so on? Do you have a quiet room available for group administration of questionnaires or for focus groups? Do you have a printer to make copies of questionnaires in-house?

3. Are language, literacy, physical stamina, or cognitive impairments likely to be a problem for your clientele in terms of completing questionnaires or taking part in fitness assessments? Is time (before, during, or after class) likely to be a factor in assessment?

4. Using your list of client outcomes, go back to the section on fitness, performance, and self-report scales and highlight the tools that may be of interest to your program.

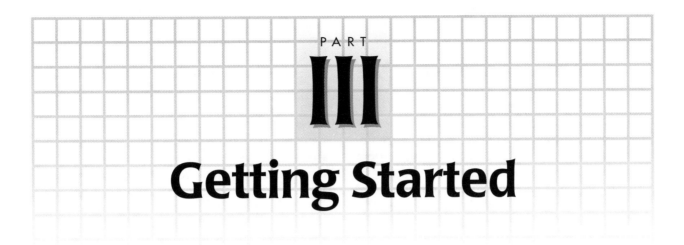

III

Getting Started

By working through the exercises at the end of chapters 1 through 5, you have laid the groundwork for evaluating your programs and have, in essence, conducted an evaluability assessment of your program.

An *evaluability assessment* is a planning process that involves

1. identifying the program's information needs;
2. clarifying and linking program activities and objectives;
3. focusing evaluation activities and setting priorities; and
4. selecting data-collection tools based on the types of information desired and considerations of feasibility, acceptability, and credibility.

The purpose of evaluability assessment is to enhance the *utilization* of evaluation. Doing the right type of evaluation at the right time, such as needs assessment in the initial planning stage or process evaluation in the operational stage, enhances the likelihood that findings will be relevant and useful for timely decision making.

At the end of chapter 1, you began by making a list of what you would like to know about your program and your participants. You identified the primary stakeholders in your program and listed the types of information each group might want to know. You began thinking about how you could use such information for modifying recruitment or program delivery to better meet the needs and expectations or your clientele. I recommended that you go through these exercises,

as well as the other chapter exercises, as a group or team (i.e., with other exercise leaders from your facility and, ideally, with representatives from other stakeholder groups).

At the end of chapter 2, you identified possible barriers that may inhibit clients from joining your program or facility, or contribute to the dropout rate. You highlighted the factors that you can do something about. You thought about how to define an absent member or program dropout. By the end of chapter 3, you had taken a close look at your current record-keeping practices. You became aware of the limitations inherent in client-satisfaction surveys and the advantages of individual over aggregate attendance records.

Part II of this book helped you focus your evaluation activities. Chapter 4 described the primary approaches to evaluation with respect to stage of planning and information sources. Recall that all types of evaluation strive to systematically collect and report credible information that is useful for timely decision making. The exercises at the end of chapter 4 had you work toward consensus on your program objectives and evaluation priorities. Templates helped you develop and clarify program objectives and construct a program logic model to guide your evaluation planning.

Chapter 5 exposed you to several ways to collect evaluation information. I recommended some practical data-collection strategies for programs doing their own needs assessments, formative, implementation, process, or outcome evaluations. At the end of the chapter, you took an inventory of your current fitness assessment protocols, your program's available fitness assessment equipment and personnel, and the characteristics of your clientele that may affect tool selection.

In part III, chapter 6 picks up where chapter 5 left off and helps you start collecting basic evaluation information. I begin by showing you how to obtain participant consent for your evaluation projects. Because most of your programs are up and running, process and outcome evaluation will likely be your priorities. Chapter 6 shows you how to profile your clientele, track participation rates, contact and assess dropouts, and assess client outcomes. You can modify the tools provided to suit your program and clientele.

Focus groups are one of the best strategies for obtaining the input of potential clients if you are considering offering new services or expanding your client base (needs assessment and formative evaluation) and for obtaining detailed feedback from current clients (process evaluation). Chapter 6 takes you through each step of planning and conducting focus groups and provides example protocols and scripts to use in evaluating exercise programs.

Chapter 7 shows you what to do with the evaluation information you collect. Step-by-step, I show you how to manage, analyze, interpret, use, and present evaluation information. I provide templates to illustrate data coding, entry, analyses, and reports. I show you how to interpret and display evaluation findings. Most important, I show you how evaluation findings can help you make decisions regarding program modification or expansion.

Collecting Basic Evaluation Information

If your programs are up and running, process and outcome evaluation are your priorities. Programs that wish to expand their client base, however, should also consider needs assessment to obtain the input of potential new clients. Programs developing new services or recruitment strategies should do formative evaluation to test draft materials.

Although published measures are available for assessing potential client outcomes (as noted in chapter 5), you will need to develop your own forms to obtain client-background information and protocols for recording participation, attendance, or usage and for contacting and assessing absent members. To help you get started, this chapter contains examples of consent forms, a client-background questionnaire, a follow-up questionnaire, suggestions for tracking participation rates, and a prototype for contacting and assessing absent members and dropouts. You can easily modify these tools for your program and clientele.

If you plan on using mail or telephone surveys of potential clients, you will need to develop survey tools based on what you what to find out. You'll need to tailor surveys for needs assessment and formative evaluation purposes to your specific program and the target group you wish to attract. However, for obtaining the input of potential clients for needs assessment and formative evaluation, I recommend focus groups over surveys. Similarly, focus groups are the best way to obtain detailed feedback and suggestions from current clients (for process evaluation). This chapter presents a 12-step approach to conducting your focus groups and provides examples of focus group protocols and scripts used in evaluating exercise programs.

Regardless of which published measures you select for outcome evaluation, you still need to decide when to conduct pre- and postassessments and how many clients you will need to assess. This chapter provides guidelines for assessing client outcomes.

Before you start on specific evaluation projects, however, you'll need to obtain the consent of those individuals you'll be asking to participate in your evaluation projects.

Obtaining Participant Consent

Most fitness programs and facilities secure liability waivers and emergency medical authorizations before allowing participation. Many programs also obtain client consent when conducting maximal or submaximal aerobic testing during screening or fitness appraisals. Sample forms are available in CSEP's 1996 appraisal manual and ACSM's (1997a) guidelines for health-fitness facilities. Similarly, programs should obtain written consent before collecting any information for evaluation purposes. Guidelines for obtaining client consent are as follows:

1. Clients are fully informed.

2. Clients have the opportunity to ask questions and receive clarification.

3. Clients are able to withdraw from the assessment without penalty or jeopardy.

4. You obtain permission before assessment begins.

Fully informed means that clients understand precisely what you are asking of them, how long it will take, what possible risks or adverse effects are involved, and what you will do with the information collected.

Worksheets 6.1 through 6.3 and 6.6 through 6.8 provide some prototype consent forms that you can adapt for your evaluation projects. Recall that you can aggregate information from individual fitness appraisals across clients for evaluation purposes. However, you need to inform clients that you will use the information for multiple purposes as worksheet 6.1 shows. In this sample consent for assessment form, note that clients are assured their participation is voluntary, and whether or not they complete the assessments will in no way affect the services they receive now or in the future.

I recommend developing separate consent forms for each assessment phase. For instance, worksheet 6.2 is designed to secure client con-

sent for follow-up assessment. If you have time-limited programs or sessions and want to assess maintenance of lifestyle changes, such as weight, smoking cessation, and dietary or exercise practices, you will need to ask clients to return to the facility, mail follow-up questionnaires to them, or interview them over the phone. Physical assessments will require that they return to your center, unless the program is taking place in a workplace or congregate residence, or unless you have the resources to conduct such assessments in their homes.

You may incorporate the guidelines in these worksheets into your existing membership contract or consent forms. Keep in mind that if you wish to contact clients in the future (for any purpose, including client-satisfaction questionnaires), obtain their permission for contact *beforehand*. Worksheet 6.3, for example, secures permission for follow-up contact of clients who have been absent from the program for an extended period.

Worksheet 6.1
Consent Form for Assessments

We would like you to do a walking test, a balance test, and a flexibility test that should take approximately 20 minutes. An assessor will be by your side for safety. Then we will ask you to complete two short questionnaires (to obtain background information and assess the way you feel) that should take no more than 20 minutes.

Your participation is totally voluntary and in no way will affect the services you now receive or may receive in the future. You may stop the tests at any time or choose not to complete one or both questionnaires.

We will keep the information from these assessments secure and confidential. We will use results to develop your personal exercise plan and monitor your progress in the program. We will also use results for evaluation purposes to provide a general description of the men and women taking part in this program. We will summarize information from these assessments and attendance records and report them as group findings. We will not identify individuals in evaluation reports. Do you have any questions?

- -

Consent Form

You have explained the purposes of these assessments to my satisfaction, and I have had the opportunity to ask questions. I will receive a copy of this consent to participate form. If I have any questions or concerns arising from these assessments, I should contact _____.

Participant's name (please print) _____

Participant's signature _____ Date _____

Worksheet 6.2
Consent Form for Follow-Up Assessment

We would like permission to contact you for a follow-up assessment approximately ___ months after you finish your session. We will be contacting you by phone to arrange a convenient time for you to return to our center (facility or clinic) to undergo the same assessments you have completed today, with the exception of the background questionnaire. We will substitute a short checklist concerning current behaviors for the background form.

We will compare information from follow-up assessments to the initial assessments to examine changes. Also, we will summarize and report information by group findings; we will not identify individuals in evaluation reports. We will keep these sheets secure. We will not give your name and phone number to anyone or use them for any purpose apart from this evaluation project. Do you have any questions?

Consent Form

You have explained the purpose of the follow-up assessment to my satisfaction, and I have had the opportunity to ask questions. By signing below, I give the program permission to contact me by telephone to arrange a possible time to return to the center for follow-up assessment. I understand that I may not agree at that time, and should I decline, you will make no further contact and will destroy this form.

Printed name_____   Phone number_____

Signature_____   Date_____

Best times to call _____morning _____afternoon _____early evening

Client Confidentiality

In each sample consent form, assure clients that you will keep the information they provide *confidential*. The issue is how your program meets this assurance.

Fitness facilities and programs routinely obtain a great deal of personal information on their clients or members. For payment purposes, programs not only have clients' names, addresses, and phone numbers, but also have credit card or bank account numbers (for preauthorized payment plans). Emergency contact information, which may be on a separate form or included in a registration form, often requests the names and phone numbers of physicians and family members. Then there are medical history forms. Even if programs do not conduct fitness appraisals or collect additional information for evaluation purposes, they still have the responsibility to protect all personal client information.

Securing Files

If you keep client information—payment authorizations, liability waivers, assessment summaries, emergency contacts—manually in individual file folders, secure the files in locked filing cabinets. Only program personnel should have access to these cabinets. Establish and follow specific access procedures as to which personnel have authorization and for what purposes. Establish similar procedures for client information stored on computer. You can use restricted passwords for designated personnel to access specific types of client information.

As you add fitness appraisals and other evaluation measures, such as background questionnaires, outcome measures, and so on, to your customized client-information system, you increase the amount of information that you must keep secure. Chapter 7 addresses in detail how to manage this information. For now, what is important is that you consider the issue of client confidentiality.

Worksheet 6.3
Consent Form for Follow-Up Contact

We are asking your permission to allow us to contact you by telephone if you should choose to leave the program (club) or be absent from the program (club) for an extended time. We would like to know whether you plan to return to the program (club) at a future date. Because your well-being is important to us, we would like to know how you are doing. To serve our members better, including you, it is important for us to know why people leave and whether there is anything you think we can do to improve our services. Do you have any questions?

- -

Consent Form

You have explained the purpose of follow-up contact to my satisfaction, and I have had the opportunity to ask questions. By signing below, I give the program permission to contact me by telephone to conduct a short, 10-minute interview concerning my absence from the program and my future intentions. I understand that I may not agree at that time, and should I decline, you will make no further contact and will destroy this form. I further understand that for evaluation purposes, you will summarize the results across individuals and will never identify individuals in program reports.

Printed name_____   Phone number (or address)_____

Signature_____   Date_____

Best times to call _____morning _____afternoon _____early evening

Assigning Unique Identifiers

Assigning a unique identifier to each client or member is a good strategy for ensuring confidentiality and linking client information. As each client enters your facility or program, assign him or her an identification number (ID #) or code. For instance, person A joins the program on January 1, 2001. Their ID # would be 01/01/01/01 (mm/dd/yy/entry). Person B also joins later the same day. His or her ID # would be 01/01/01/02. This system allows up to 99 people to join your club or program on the same day—each person with a unique identifier.

You can use other identification systems also, such as making client birth dates part of the identifier (the potential problem is that clients may have the same birth dates). You can also use a combination of alpha (letter) and numeric codes, such as client initials combined with birth date and month (e.g., AM/02/09) or letter codes for type of membership, such as G for Gold or full-facility access. Such systems, however, are more complex and vulnerable to duplication. I recommend the first system described above. An added advantage is that such a system allows you to track members easily according to when they first registered for your program.

The Centre for Activity and Ageing assigns a unique identifier to each participant based on the date and order of initial registration. The Centre has over a dozen on-site exercise programs and enters all registrants into their database. We examined data collected over a three-year period on a database of 670 registrants to look at patterns of attendance, transfers between classes, and long-term adherence (Ecclestone, Myers, and Patterson 1998). Such an examination was more feasible due to having unique identifiers for each registrant. For instance, we were able see how long clients stayed in a program (date class began, together with date clients registered and attendance records). We were also able to accurately estimate dropout rates by identifying people registered in more than one program and to track movement patterns between classes.

In addition to facilitating client tracking, unique identifiers help protect client confidentiality. You can put identifiers, rather than names, directly on medical forms, background questionnaires, or fitness appraisal summary sheets, or later substitute them for names when you file or enter the information into the computer database. Keep in mind that you will defeat your purpose (protecting client information such as fitness appraisal results with an ID #) if you store such information in the same files folders as consent forms, waivers, or other pieces of information containing the client's name. A secured master list can be used to link client unique identifiers to their names, addresses, and phone numbers.

As noted in chapter 3, you must keep client-satisfaction surveys (comment or suggestion cards) anonymous or clients are unlikely to fill them out. This is one problem of such surveys—there is no way to link the information to client characteristics, attendance patterns, and so on.

Another situation in which you need to take special precautions to protect anonymity is when focus group participants are still program clients. Reassure participants that any feedback they provide on the program will in no way jeopardize either current or future services received. As you will see in the discussion of focus groups, there are special consent forms for this purpose (worksheets 6.6 through 6.8).

Profiling Your Clientele

A short background questionnaire can serve several purposes. When conducting process and outcome evaluation projects, it is important to document the extent to which your samples are *representative* of your overall program clientele. Programs should be collecting background information on each and every new client or member.

Most programs have registration forms. Many have medical history forms. As noted in chapter 3, however, programs often cannot provide more than a vague description or crude age and gender breakdown of their clientele. Besides gender and age, what else do you want to know about your clientele?

Their level of education or income

How physically active they are when they join your program or facility

Whether they are members at other fitness facilities or clubs

How far away they live and how they get to the program

Their health practices, such as smoking

A carefully designed background questionnaire customized for your program can provide valuable data for

- profiling your clientele,
- determining whether you are reaching your intended audience,
- determining whether your client profile changes over time,
- comparing your clientele to similar sectors of the fitness industry,
- determining the types of clients who are the most frequent users of various classes or facility sections,
- comparing continuing versus discontinuing clients,
- determining whether your evaluation samples are representative, and
- determining which types of clients benefit most.

Published, validated, paper-and-pencil measures for examining physical activity level do exist; however, they tend to be time consuming for clients to complete and difficult for administrators to code and score. There are also numerous published health and functional status assessment questionnaires, some of which I described in chapter 5. However, there is no single published tool that comprehensively captures everything you might want to profile about your clients.

Worksheet 6.4 shows a prototype background questionnaire to get you started. Let's look at this prototype and review why you would select certain questions and response formats. As we go through this exercise, think about what you want to know about your clients.

Part A Tell Us About Yourself

General background information is the most important section for profiling your clientele. All programs should collect information on clients' gender (question 1) and age (question 2).

Worksheet 6.4
Prototype Background Questionnaire

Name or ID _____ Date completed _____

Part A

Tell us about yourself.

1. Are you ____ **male** or ___ **female?**
2. What is your **date of birth?** _____ month _____ day _____ year
3. Have you **completed high school?** ____ no ____ yes   **College?** ____ no ____ yes
4. Are you **currently employed** ___ full time ___ part time ___ self-employed ___ between jobs
   ___ a homemaker or caretaker ___ a student ___ semiretired ___ fully retired?
5. How would you describe your **financial situation?** (Choose one.)

   ___ I can meet my needs and still have enough money left to do **most** things I want.

   ___ I have enough money to do **many** things I want if I **budget carefully.**

   ___ I have enough to meet my needs but have **little left for extras.**

   ___ I can barely meet my needs and have **nothing left for extras.**

Part B

Tell us about your health.

6. In **general**, how would you describe your **current, overall state of health?** (Check one.)
   ___ excellent ___ good   ___ fair ___ poor
7. Are you a current, regular **smoker?** ___ no ___ yes (Do you want to quit? ___ no ___ yes)
8. Do you consider yourself overweight _____ underweight _____ at the right weight ____?
9. Are you a frequent **dieter?** ___ no ___ yes
10. Have you ever been **diagnosed by a health professional** as having any of the following?
    (Check all that apply.)   **Yes**

    Heart trouble   ____

    Chronic asthma, emphysema, or bronchitis   ____

    Diabetes   ____

    Osteoporosis   ____

    Arthritis   ____

    High blood pressure   ____

    High cholesterol   ____

    Back problems   ____

    Foot problems   ____

    Allergies (including hay fever and sinus problems)   ____

    Trouble hearing   ____

    Trouble seeing   ____

    Other health problems   ____

    What are they? _____.

11. Are you currently on any **prescribed medications?** ___ no (Go to next question.) ___ yes
    If yes, **what is the medication(s) for** (for example, heart or arthritis)?

    _____

12. Do you use
    prescription eye glasses?   ___ no ___ yes   a hearing aid? ___ no ___ yes
    a foot orthotic?   ___ no ___ yes   a walking aid? ___ no ___ yes

13. Are you **currently limited** in the type or amount of *physical* activity (work or leisure) you
    can do because of an illness, injury, or disability?
    ___ no (Go to next question.)
    ___ yes, because of a **temporary** illness or injury (example: flu, fracture, sprain)
    Specify_____
    ___ yes, because of a **long-term** illness, injury, or disability (example: diabetes, arthritis,
    chronic foot, back or joint problems, heart disease)
    Specify_____

Part C

Now, tell us about your current activities.

14. About how many **hours on a weekday** (Monday to Friday) do you spend relaxing or
    doing leisure activities you enjoy? _____ hours

15. What do you usually do in your **leisure time?**

    Time for yourself   **With other people**
    _____   _____
    _____   _____

16. Do you consider yourself to be a **physically active** person **now?**
    ___ very much so   ___ somewhat   ___ not really

17. Would you say you have **always** been a **physically active** person?
    ___ yes, all my life   ___ off and on   ___ not really

18. To what extent is exercising or playing sports **currently an important part** of your
    regular routine? (Circle number.)

1	2	3	4	5
Not at all important		Moderately important		Extremely important

19. Are you **currently enrolled** in any organized physical activity **classes** or **groups** that
    meet regularly **apart from this class?** ___ no __ yes

20. Do you do any **other types** of regular physical activity (at least once a week) besides
    organized exercise classes (for example: home exercise, brisk walking, swimming, biking,
    calisthenics, exercise equipment)? ___ no ___ yes

21. Do you participate in any **sports** regularly (at least once a week) either year-round or
    during a particular season, for example, tennis, golf, baseball, skiing? ___ no ___ yes

22. Taking all these activities (exercise classes, sports, walking, etc.) into consideration, **how
    many days in an average week do you accumulate 30 minutes or more of
    moderate intensity physical activity** (equivalent to a brisk walk)? _____ days a week

23. What are your **preferred times** for exercising or playing sports?
   a. ___ weekdays   ___ weekends   ___ both
   b. ___ early morning   ___ mid to late morning   ___ early afternoon
      ___ mid to late afternoon   ___ early evening   ___ late evening
24. Does your **doctor ever inquire** about whether you exercise?
   ___ no ___ yes   ___ Not applicable, I don't see a doctor annually.
25. Do you **tell your doctor** about your exercise?   ___ no ___ yes
26. To what extent are you **encouraged** and **supported** to be physically active?

	Very much so	Somewhat	Not at all
a. By family	_____	_____	_____
b. By friends	_____	_____	_____
c. By doctor	_____	_____	_____
d. Self-motivated	_____	_____	_____

Part D

Finally, please answer a few questions about this program.

27. How did you **hear about** *this* class or program?

_____

28. Do you **know anyone** in this class or program? ___ no ___ yes
29. What are your **personal reasons** for coming to *this* class or program?

_____
_____

30. Have you **previously participated** in this or a similar type of exercise class?
   ___ no ___ yes, this class   ___ yes, a similar class
31. How **sure** are you that you will be **able to do** the exercises in this class or program
   without becoming overly fatigued, tired, or short of breath? (Circle number.)

0	1	2	3	4
Very sure (no problem)	Pretty sure	Not very sure (may be too much)	Know I couldn't	Don't know (never tried it before)

32. Do you have any **reservations or concerns** about taking this class? (Check all that
   apply.)
   ____ No.
   ____ I may not have the skills or be able to keep up.
   ____ I may not be able to schedule the time to attend all classes.
   ____ I may have transportation problems.
   ____ Other concerns (specify) _____
   _____

Thank you for completing this background questionnaire. The information provided will assist the instructors in tailoring the program to the needs and interests of you and your fellow participants. If you found any sections unclear, please bring this to the attention of your instructor.

Please note: Your instructor may ask you to complete some additional short forms. If so, they will be attached to this package. Once again, ask your instructor if anything is unclear.

Birth date is more accurate than asking a person's age (the latter must be linked to date of questionnaire completion).

Education, employment, and financial questions (3 to 5) are optional, depending on what you want to know about your clientele. As noted in chapter 2, accessibility due to transportation or finances may be barriers to participation. People who are more educated are likely to be physically active. People who have not finished high school are likely to have difficulty reading program materials. There are many different ways of obtaining information on education level (such as years of schooling, highest degree attained), employment, or income. We have found that whether clients completed high school is a good predictor of whether they are likely to be physically active or sedentary (Myers et al. in press).

Inquiring about a person's income is often a sensitive issue, because people do not like to divulge their incomes. Income is also complex—gross versus net (after tax) income, income from various sources, single versus dual incomes, and so on. As Grantham et al. (1998) note, money spent on exercise equipment, clothing, or club fees for most people comes out of their discretionary income. Question 5 illustrates a good way to get at clients' perceived ability to pay for extras, such as fitness classes, and most people do not mind answering this type of question.

Part B Tell Us About Your Health

Part B illustrates the types of questions that you can use to get at health perceptions, practices, and problems. Many health surveys have used question 6, and it is a good indicator of overall perceived health status. Questions 7 through 9 are simple ways to get at smoking and dieting patterns. Questions 10 through 12 address specific health problems, medication use, and use of assistive devices. Unlike glasses, hearing aids are not always visible. Exercise instructors should be aware of which participants have vision and hearing problems. Question 13 comes from a national fitness survey conducted in Canada (Stephens and Craig 1990) and is an excellent single question for getting at perceived physical limitations.

Part C Tell Us About Your Current Activities

Part C examines leisure time and preferred activities (questions 14 and 15); perceived level and importance of physical activity (16 through 18); current activities, such as classes, sports, and unstructured activities (19 through 21); preferred times for exercising or sports (23); and perceived support to exercise (24 through 26).

Question 22 is a crude way of estimating normal level of physical activity with respect to number of days a week the respondent accumulates 30 minutes or more of moderate-intensity physical activity. This question is based on the recommendation of Pate et al. (1995) and endorsed by the Surgeon General (United States Department of Health and Human Services 1996) for the general public (see chapter 1). The precision and complexity inherent in published physical activity questionnaires used for research purposes is unnecessary for most programs. As an alternative to question 22, you could use the three questions taken from the CSEP fitness appraisal manual listed on p. 73. If you do fitness appraisals on new clients, you will have a more objective measure of their actual fitness. Self-report questions, such as questions 19 to 22, however, are necessary to determine how people get their exercise.

Part D A Few Questions About This Program

Part D solicits information concerning how clients heard about the class or program (27), whether they know anyone in the class (28), and personal reasons for coming to the class or program (29). When aggregated across clients, such information can be useful in examining the reach of your advertisement strategies. Recall from chapter 2 that word of mouth is the greatest source for generating new clients.

Chapter 2 discusses the importance of outcome expectations and self-efficacy expectations regarding exercise adoption and adherence. Chapter 5 shows you some published self-efficacy tools and how you need to tailor these to the specific exercise regimen. Question 29 gets at each client's outcome expectations in terms of their personal reasons for joining. Question 30 examines their prior experience participating in this type of class or regimen. Question 31 is a simple self-efficacy question pertaining to the specific class or program in question. The final question (32) examines reservations or concerns about taking the class. Any of these questions may be helpful in predicting exercise adherence across your clientele. Clients with no prior experience, low self-confidence, and reservations about keeping up with the class are more likely to drop out.

Adapt this template to your needs by deleting or adding questions or parts. If you work with older clientele, use a large font (14 point versus 12 point). Bear in mind that this prototype was designed to obtain information from *new clients* when they first join the program or facility. If you choose to administer such a questionnaire to *current clients*, omit or modify some questions in parts C and D as appropriate, because they have already been participating in the program.

Similarly, if you wish to obtain background information on evaluation project samples for descriptive purposes, you can modify this form accordingly. Keep it short and use close-ended or checklist response formats (versus open-ended questions) as much as possible. Gender is readily observable, but you still may wish to solicit this information via a checklist to describe your sample in terms of gender breakdowns by age. Sample characteristics, as well as experience with the program in question (such as length of time in the class), are the types of information typically assessed through a short questionnaire administered at the end of a focus group session, at the end of a survey, or in conjunction with an outcome evaluation study.

All programs should obtain some demographic, health, and activity information to accurately profile or describe their clientele. The specific information you choose to collect depends on whether you plan to assess new clients, current clients, or samples (e.g., focus group participants). Modify your background questionnaires according to your purpose. Chapter 7 shows you how to code, analyze, interpret, and use the information you gather from such questionnaires.

Tracking Participation Rates

In addition to background information, attendance or participation rates are necessary to pro-
file frequent versus infrequent users of your programs or services and to compare continued users versus dropouts for process evaluation purposes. Outcome evaluation also requires information on participation rates. The basic assumption is that clients who attend exercise classes more often, or are more compliant with a prescribed exercise regimen, achieve better outcomes, such as weight loss or improved fitness. Thus, participation rates are critical for both process and outcome evaluation.

Chapter 3 provides formulas for determining average length of membership and attrition rates across all the clients in your program. Remember to take attendance individually for every client on a class-by-class basis. As shown in chapter 3, you can readily calculate aggregate or average usage rates from individual attendance records (total the number who attended, divide by the number of sessions, and multiply by 100). However, you cannot determine individual participation rates and patterns from aggregate data!

If the exercise regimen does not involve a class (e.g., a home exercise program), give each client a daily exercise log or diary to determine exercise participation rates, and encourage him or her to fill it out. You can use a similar strategy to record individual workouts. For instance, each time members use the weight room, they could pull their logs from a filing cabinet in the room and record the date, time (in and out), and the number of repetitions (and weight settings) at each station. Similarly, swimmers could pull their logs from a file box in the locker room adjacent to the pool and record the date and duration of each swim, number of laps, or other exercises in the pool. A fitness instructor should carefully go through exercise logs with each person during their orientation session. Incentives, such as T-shirts, may increase compliance with log completion. If you make self-monitoring an integral part of the exercise regimen at the beginning, clients are more likely to be compliant.

Grantham et al. (1998) argue that monitoring usage rates to determine peak periods (days of the week, times of the day) can be useful for guiding staffing and equipment purchases. In addition, you can use the data for evaluation purposes. Understandably, tracking participation rates is more complicated for large fitness facilities with multiple classes and services. Class or attendance recording is straightforward. Monitoring pool use (outside aquafitness classes) and the use of treadmills, weights, and other equipment is not as easy.

Technology, such as computerized check-in systems, bar code scanners, or treadmills that require cards to operate, can greatly facilitate the tracking process. However, high technology is not essential. Personal fitness logs or diaries are good strategies for self-monitoring, and if you ask individuals to submit their logs regularly (say monthly), you can use them to calculate participation rates.

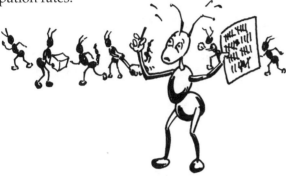

If large facilities simply want to get an overall sense of member use, they may wish to set up a defined evaluation period to obtain a snapshot of their club in action. In advance of the evaluation period, perhaps use posters to remind members to bring their membership cards, or you could give members a card to tag to their shirt as they enter the facility during this period. You could color code the type of membership using dots (e.g., gold for full-facility use, red for squash, green for tennis, etc.). Plan sampling periods (times of day and areas) in advance. During the evaluation period, staff would enter designated areas of the facility for specified time periods (say 15-minute blocks) and record the number of users by membership number, category (according to their tags), and gender (which is easily observed).

Contacting and Assessing Absentees

As Grantham et al. (1998) note, it is important for every fitness facility and program to flag absent or inactive members and encourage such members to resume active participation *before* they become dropouts. To do so, each program should develop and implement a standardized protocol for contacting and assessing absent members.

First, you need to decide what constitutes an absent or inactive member. You could use gate or sign-in records to flag members who have not been to the club for a specified period (e.g., one month) or class attendance sheets to identify participants who have missed a specified number of consecutive sessions (e.g., 12 sessions). Then, you need to decide how to contact absent members and the protocol for the contact.

If an exercise class is small and has only one instructor, it is likely that the instructor will notice that a participant is absent, particularly if that participant has been a regular attendee. Often the instructor informally inquires about the participant's absence by asking someone else in the class, "Have you seen John? Is he okay?" If coparticipants relay the instructor's message of concern and caring to the absent member, this could serve as a motivator for coming back to the class.

A more formal and standardized protocol, however, is necessary to obtain information on absent clients for evaluation purposes. For instance, you could send letters expressing concern and encouragement to all absent clients after a specified period of absence. Letters, however, are impersonal and unlikely to be as effective as a telephone call. Also, unless you enclose a questionnaire survey with the letter, you will not learn reasons for absence.

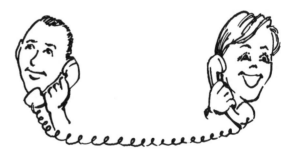

Wankel and Thompson (1977) have demonstrated that personal phone calls from staff lasting only five minutes can increase resumption rate. Many fitness clubs have a standard practice of calling absent or inactive members. Usually, the purposes of these phone calls are twofold: (a) to encourage members to resume activity, and (b) to determine intention to pay outstanding or late fees or dues. Such phone calls could also serve an important third purpose—to obtain information on reasons for absence or dropout.

Worksheet 6.5
Prototype for Contacting Absentees

"Hello Mrs./Ms./Mr./Dr. _____. This is _____ calling from _____. We haven't seen you at _____ since _____ and were worried about you." Allow the person time to give you his or her reasons for absence.

Probe 1. If the person volunteers that they or a family member have been injured or ill, respond appropriately: *"I am sorry to hear that. I hope it is not too serious (or I hope you or they are feeling better)."*
Record nature of illness/injury to participant _____
or significant other _____ and relationship _____.

Probe 2. If the person does not volunteer a reason, gently inquire as to reasons for absence. *"We miss you at the program (class, club) and wondered if there was anything we could do to help you resume your exercise. Was the class time inconvenient for you? Was it something else about the program or the facility that did not meet your needs or expectations?"*
Record reasons for absence: _____
_____

Probe 3. If the client suggests he or she may return, then probe further.
"So you think you may be able to return by _____." (Record projected time.)
"Would it be okay if we call you again around that time?" ___no ___ yes
Conclude by thanking him or her for taking the time to talk with you, and express your best wishes.
Record date _____ and _____ time of contact.
Interviewer's comments _____
_____

Worksheet 6.5 provides a prototype for contacting absentees, encouraging resumption, and obtaining information on reasons for absence and intentions to resume activity. Similar to the other prototypes contained in this book, you can modify this example to suit your clientele and your needs for information. For instance, if you address relapse planning with each client during their initial appraisal, you could refer to this information during the follow-up contact.

Recall that you should obtain consent for follow-up contact while clients are in the program, preferably when they first join (refer to worksheet 6.3). Keep in mind that your protocol should be standardized, or consistent:

1. Establish your criteria for absenteeism.
2. Use the same calling and callback procedures (times of day and number of attempts).
3. Follow the same script and prompts for all calls.

There are a few ways you can learn more about your absent members and dropouts. First, you can try to get such clients to attend focus groups. Although this strategy may be feasible with certain groups, such as the company employees in the corporate fitness scenario, it will be difficult to get people who have left the club or program to return for focus groups. Dissatisfied or disinterested clients are more likely to consent to a short telephone interview.

For the reasons above, a structured telephone contact protocol is preferred over a letter and survey questionnaire. If you are unable to contact absent members by phone, and this likely will be the case for at least some clients, you still have a fallback for profiling dropouts. Although you will not be able to ascertain reasons for absence or dropout, you still can develop a profile of dropout characteristics through information from the background questionnaires they completed at program entry.

Obtaining Client Feedback Through Focus Groups

Use focus groups to obtain in-depth feedback from several people at the same time. In contrast to individual interviews, the dynamic nature of group discussions encourages interaction and debate. Individual opinions may shift during the course of the discussion, similar to how people's opinions are influenced in life (Krueger 1994). For these reasons, focus groups have been used by market researchers to obtain consumer input on new products or services and feedback concerning existing products or services.

Increasingly, focus groups are being used to develop and evaluate nonprofit programs. It has taken a while for this methodology to achieve credibility outside the marketing field because people tend to be less familiar and comfortable with nonnumerical data (Krueger 1994). Although human services acknowledge the importance of the consumer's point of view, the tendency has been to rely on consumer satisfaction surveys. Such surveys are easy to develop and tailor to the service in question, easy for clients to complete, and easy to score. Moreover, such surveys yield numerical data! Unfortunately, consumer satisfaction surveys do not yield a great deal of insight about why clients are satisfied or dissatisfied or how programs can better meet client expectations.

Like many evaluators, I have become an enthusiastic user and advocate of the focus group strategy (cf. Krueger 1994; Morgan 1993). You do *not* have to be a professional evaluator to become adept at conducting focus groups. However, you do need to carefully follow specific guidelines to plan and execute successful focus groups that yield credible and useful information for program decision making. This section outlines, in 12 steps (shown in figure 6.1), what is involved and what resources are required to get the most out of your focus group data.

Step 1 Decide on the Purpose of Your Focus Group

All too often we are brought together in groups or committees in our workplaces for meetings. Have you ever felt that many committees you are on or the multiple meetings you attend are a waste of time? The reason is probably that the pur-

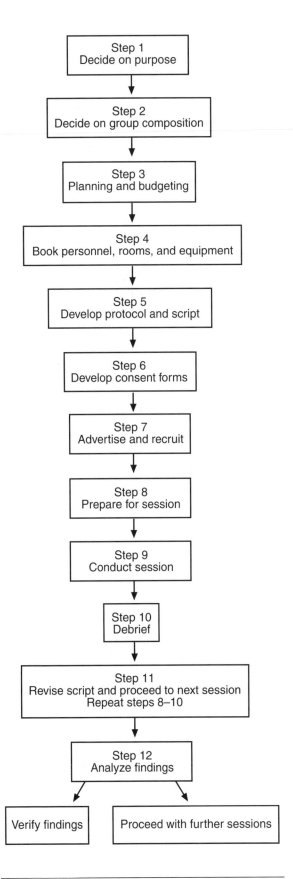

Figure 6.1 A 12-step approach to conducting focus groups.

pose or mandate of the group is unclear or overwhelming. Poor leadership often further contributes to the frustration many of us experience with group meetings (Krueger 1994).

A *focus group* is a special type of group discussion with respect to purpose, composition, and procedures. The purpose of focus groups is to obtain "perceptions on a defined area of interest in a permissive, nonthreatening environment" (Krueger 1994, 6). Participants are brought together who share characteristics or experiences (as potential consumers, current consumers, or former consumers) relevant to the topic of discussion. Focus groups are carefully assembled to avoid power struggles (in contrast to most workplace meetings). Procedures are established in advance and ground rules are communicated at the beginning of each session to encourage everyone to contribute and to avoid a few people dominating the conversation. Using a carefully developed and structured script, the facilitator keeps the discussion on track. Again, think of meetings in which there is no agenda, or no one sticks to the agenda. Often the meeting time is over before pressing issues ever get discussed, and these issues get tabled for the next meeting.

Focus groups are the preferred strategy for obtaining input from potential consumers in needs assessment and are by far the best strategy for conducting formative evaluation. Because most of your programs are probably operational, process and outcome evaluation are likely to be on top of your evaluation priority list. Although you should not use focus groups as the primary strategy for outcome evaluation, they can be useful for establishing meaningful client-outcome objectives and selecting suitable measures. In this regard, you could use focus groups to obtain client perceptions concerning both positive and adverse program effects.

Recall that the director in scenario 1 (p. 6) wanted to know why only half of the 20 employees continued coming to the aerobics class. The satisfaction survey after the first month indicated high satisfaction by those who were in class that day. To obtain more in-depth feedback for process evaluation, it would be useful to conduct focus groups with employees who continued with the class for several months (what kept them coming back?). It would also be useful to conduct focus groups with employees who started but quit the aerobics class (why did they stop coming?). Similarly, it would be informative to explore why other employees chose not to sign up for the aerobics program (why didn't they join?).

Once you have determined the information you want from your focus group—the purpose of the evaluation project—you can move to step 2.

Step 2 Decide on Group Composition

Each focus group should include a minimum of 6 and a maximum of 12 participants (Krueger 1994; Mertens 1998; Morgan 1993). If there are fewer than 6, there is more pressure on each person to continue the discussion. As the size of the group increases, participants have less opportunity to express their viewpoints. The typical duration of a focus group session is 60 to 90 minutes. However, focus group sessions can last up to two hours. When working with certain populations, such as injured workers or frail, older adults, it is particularly important—and more effective—to keep the session short (60 minutes or less).

I recommend at least two focus groups for each evaluation project, but you may need up to six or eight, depending on the feedback and trends you see in the first two sessions (Krueger 1994; Mertens 1998). You should make some decisions on group mix or composition in advance, before recruitment (as described below based on desired representativeness). Analyzing the findings from the first two sessions, however, is necessary to determine whether there is sufficient diversity of responses and whether the findings reach *saturation*. Saturation means that the themes that emerge from the discussions become repetitive, and you are likely to gain little by conducting more groups.

Desired representativeness relates to the purpose of the evaluation project. Decide on whose viewpoints you want to include in your focus groups. For needs assessment and formative evaluation, focus group participants should be representative with respect to the characteristics that define your intended audience. For instance, scenario 2 (p. 7) targets women working in the textile plant. The health educator needs to further decide whether she wants her focus groups to include women from different ethnic groups, women with and without families, and so on. In scenario 3 (p. 7), the YMCA manager was particularly interested in whether a new Tai Chi program would appeal to both older and younger members. In this case, member age would be the most important criteria for selecting focus group participants.

For process evaluation, focus group participants should be representative of your clientele. If roughly half of your clients are female, then you should invite both genders to participate. It is important, however, that focus group participants do not perceive themselves to be in the minority. For instance, if you wish to represent women's viewpoints, but only a handful of your clients are women, then make sure your focus groups include at least one-third women (2 of 6 or 4 of 12 participants). It will be impossible to represent all or even several demographic characteristics (age, gender, education level, income, occupation, race or ethnicity, area of residence, etc.) in a single group, so you must carefully decide what are the most important one or two characteristics regarding group composition (e.g., age and gender or gender and ethnicity).

Although you want to represent a diversity of viewpoints in each group, be careful not to mix participants likely to have radically different perspectives or power relationships. For instance, in our evaluation of the HeartMobile program, we conducted separate focus groups with managerial and frontline workers (Gray and Myers 1997). Similarly, we conducted separate focus groups with the retired men's and women's associations, because they had chosen to form their own exercise classes and we wanted to know why, from their different perspectives.

Although participants may differ on one or two characteristics, such as length of time in the program, each group should be fairly *homogeneous* (similar) with respect to program experience. For instance, in the corporate fitness scenario, it would be wise to conduct three separate focus groups: with ongoing participants, with dropouts, and with abstainers (employees who never signed up for the class). In this scenario, the number of groups will be limited by the one class (20 signed up, half continued) and small company size (100 employees in total). Although there are 80 nonjoiners to sample from, there are only 10 continued participants and 10 dropouts.

Commercial marketers never mix current users of the product or service with nonusers or with former users. Also, as a rule, marketers recruit participants who do not know each other. The reasoning is that people who are related, work together, or interact socially are more likely to have similar views and agree with each other. When recruiting potential program consumers, it is usually possible to get focus group participants who do not know one another. In large fitness facilities or work sites, it may also be possible to assemble groups of people who are not acquainted (for instance, to examine whether people would be interested in a new program or willing to pay increased fees for additional services). The smaller the facility or work site, such as the software company with 100 employees in scenario 1, the less likely that people will not know each other. For process evaluation purposes, however, the purpose of the focus group is to examine participant experiences concerning the program in question. In this case, familiarity with the program and with each other is a desirable feature of focus group composition.

Step 3 Planning and Budgeting

After deciding on the purpose and the desired composition of your focus groups, you need to plan and budget your project. The primary categories to consider are

1. personnel;
2. space, equipment, and supplies;
3. advertising strategy and costs; and
4. participant fees or incentives.

Personnel

Technically, you need only one person to conduct focus groups. Focus groups must have a leader, often referred to as the *facilitator* or *moderator*. The facilitator takes responsibility for introducing the topic and obtaining consent, establishing and enforcing ground rules, and leading participants through the discussion process. A successful focus group session is one that runs smoothly and produces lively discussion (involving all or most participants) on the topic.

Personal attributes of the facilitator are important in creating a nonthreatening, conducive environment in which participants feel comfortable enough to open up and express their opinions. The facilitator must be friendly and warm, yet be able to intervene as needed to reinforce ground rules (e.g., when everyone starts talking at the same time), prevent arguments, get the discussion back on track, and gently move the discussion from issue to issue so everything is covered in a timely manner.

The facilitator must appear neutral and should not contribute his or her opinions to the discussion. Participants are more likely to be honest and open with a neutral facilitator. For process evaluation projects, the facilitator should *not* be the program instructor, but someone more removed from the program under evaluation. The facilitator can be someone from another program in your facility or an outside consultant.

Hiring an outside facilitator is something your program may wish to consider, if your resources and the purpose of your evaluation project warrant it. A consultant could charge anywhere from $250 to $1,500 (U.S.) per day or per group, depending on credentials and expertise, how many groups he or she conducts, and whether the consultant also contracts to do the data analysis. For less than $1,000 (U.S.), you can send two or three of your personnel to a local two-day training workshop on focus groups. For about $100 (U.S.), you can purchase the six-volume *Focus Group Kit* (Morgan and Krueger 1998) from Sage Publications (805-499-9774 or **order@sagepub.com**). The guidelines in the present book may be all you need.

As is the case with becoming a good fitness instructor, becoming a good focus group leader or facilitator requires training, experience, and confidence. Facilitation skill and comfort increase with practice. As you will see, a carefully developed protocol and script are vital to conducting successful focus groups and make the facilitator's job a great deal easier.

In addition to the facilitator, it is desirable to have a second person assist in conducting focus groups. This individual is referred to as the *recorder* or *assistant*. Consultants hired as facilitators may bring their own assistant and will charge you for this service. Program personnel can also act in this role, provided he or she is perceived as neutral. The assistant's duties are to assist with preparatory activities (described shortly), act as a recorder or note taker during the session, and collaborate in the debriefing process with the facilitator immediately following the session. The recorder should not, however, contribute to or influence the discussion itself.

Space, Equipment, and Supplies

To conduct focus groups, you need a quiet room that comfortably seats up to 14 people (the 12 participants along with the facilitator and recorder). Arrange seats in a circular, U-shaped, or rectangular fashion around a table so everyone faces each other. See figure 6.2 for an illustration of a desirable seating arrangement. You can put together four card tables for this purpose, if necessary.

You can conduct focus groups without a table (chairs arranged in a circle); however, tape recording, note taking by the facilitator and recorder, and form completion by participants is much more difficult without a table.

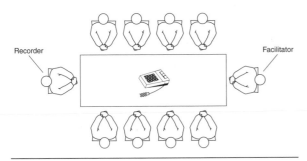

Figure 6.2 Focus group seating arrangement.

The most important piece of equipment for focus groups is a good tape recorder with a microphone that is sensitive enough to clearly pick up everyone's voice. Although the facilitator and assistant can take notes during the session, it is difficult to record everything that everyone says in a discussion that may last an hour or more.

Audiotaping the session allows the facilitator to concentrate on the process, while the recorder notes interaction styles, nonverbal gestures, and which participants are speaking during the session. The tapes from each session constitute the primary source of data, and you and others can listen to them repeatedly during the analysis phase. Transcribing costs about $150 (U.S.) per one-hour tape if you hire someone to do this. It may take three to four hours to transcribe a one-hour tape until you become proficient at transcribing. Tape recorders that include a transcribing pedal and telephone recording capabilities (useful for telephone interviews) cost between $400 and $1,000 (U.S.). Leasing such equipment is an option. Purchasing such equipment can be a good long-term investment as evaluation activities increase.

You will have to consider printing costs for participant letters of information, consent forms, and possibly a background questionnaire (or checklist). You may wish to have copies of program materials available for participants to scrutinize if this is part of the purpose of your focus groups. A flip chart is useful for recording the main ideas that emerge for summary or ranking purposes.

Advertising Strategy and Costs

If you recruit participants from outside the program (potential clients) for focus groups, you may need to consider the costs of a newspaper ad or radio announcement. A low-cost alternative is to put up posters where your target group might congregate (e.g., workplaces or commu-

nity centers). In some cases your intended target audience is readily accessible (e.g., women working at the textile plant in scenario 2 or seniors frequenting the three malls in scenario 4).

For process evaluation purposes, you will recruit volunteers from your client base. You can recruit current clients through posters, class announcements, or club newsletters. You will need to contact former clients by telephone or mail to recruit volunteers for focus groups. In any case, the recruitment ad, poster, letter, announcement, or phone call should include

1. the purpose or topic of the group discussion session;
2. eligibility criteria;
3. the location, starting time, and duration of the session;
4. incentives or compensation, if any, being offered to volunteers;
5. the sign-up process; and
6. who to call for further information about the project.

Participant Incentives

Commercial marketers pay focus group participants, anywhere from $50 (U.S.) per person for the general public to several hundred dollars for professionals such as physicians. Programs, on the other hand, are more likely to offer modest incentives such as refreshments. Select light refreshments, such as juices, soft drinks, coffee, tea, cookies, or a fruit or sandwich plate, based on the time of day and preferences. Refreshments do not have to be costly when you purchase in bulk, and they promote mingling and relaxing at the start of the session. Certificates of participation, T-shirts, or free passes to the club are other possible incentives. For some people, the opportunity to have an input concerning new or existing services may be sufficient incentive for participation.

Step 4 Book Personnel, Rooms, and Equipment

Now that you've determined the budget and planned for the focus group, you need to book the room and tape recorder, and arrange session dates and times around the schedules of the facilitator and recorder. When conducting focus groups with current clients or members, consider prescheduling sessions before or after exercise classes to save people a trip.

We have found that it is less time consuming to have volunteers sign up for preset days and times than to arrange sessions later around people's schedules. If possible, book the room for the entire day, and schedule morning, afternoon, and evening sessions to accommodate volunteer preferences. Give volunteers a choice of time periods and dates. Allow at least 45 minutes for pre- and postsession activities when booking. For instance, if you plan a one-hour discussion, book the room, equipment, and participants in two-hour blocks.

Step 5 Develop Protocol and Script

Once you have decided on the purpose of the project, group composition, recruitment strategy, and schedule, you need to develop a detailed protocol and script for conducting the focus group sessions. Remember, for each evaluation project, you should be conducting at least two focus groups. The protocol should be consistent or standardized across sessions that are part of the same project. The *protocol* outlines each step of the process for the facilitator and recorder, from before participants arrive to when they leave. Table 6.1 provides an example.

Focus group sessions require careful planning and organization ahead of time. The facilitator and recorder should arrive about 30 minutes ahead of participants to set up. Allow about 15 minutes for settling in after participants arrive. If people do not know each other, it is important to make light conversation until everyone arrives. Refreshments give people something to do while they are waiting.

Allow another 15 minutes for introductions, consent forms, and setting the ground rules. Allow 15 minutes at the end of the discussion if you plan to hand out a background checklist and follow-up consent forms for verification. If you follow this format and participants have made only a 90-minute time commitment, this will only leave 45 minutes for the discussion itself. Give participants a washroom and stretch break if they are to be there 90 minutes or longer. If you use a 90-minute tape (45 minutes per side), you can use the break as an opportunity to flip your tape over and determine how much of the script you have left to cover. Plan a break at a logical or transitional point in the discussion session.

In most focus groups, participants decide how to introduce themselves. Note that older individuals may rather be addressed by Mr. or Mrs. than by their first names. Let each person decide and fill out their own name tag. The facilitator and recorder should also wear name tags. In certain situations where anonymity is a concern, such as company employees commenting on their work site programs, consider using pseudonyms (false names). Fill two hats with fictitious male and female names and have people draw false names from the hats.

As illustrated in table 6.1, the protocol can outline introductory remarks, the consent process, ground rules, and concluding activities. You can incorporate the focus group *script*—the actual questions and probes that you will use to guide the discussion—into the protocol itself or put it on a separate sheet. As a rule, discussions begin with an icebreaker (introductory) question, and move from transitional (general) questions to key questions, and, finally, to closure (summary or wrap-up) questions. Develop only one or two questions under each category, particularly concerning the in-depth or key portion of the session.

• The *icebreaker question* should be nonthreatening, easy and quick to answer, and get everyone talking. For example, an icebreaker for a focus group for scenario 3 might be, "Let's go around the table and introduce ourselves. How long have each of you been at the club?"

• *Transitional questions* establish rapport, set the stage, and obtain general views on the topic. For instance, "The YMCA is considering introducing Tai Chi classes. What do you know about Tai Chi? What is the appeal of Tai Chi (relaxation, meditation, balance)?"

• *Key questions* generate in-depth information related to the primary purpose of the project (determined in step 1). For instance, "As members, would you like to see the YMCA start Tai Chi classes? Can you elaborate on your reasons? Would you be willing to pay an additional fee for Tai Chi classes? What are the pros and cons of having separate classes for different age groups? Do you think the YMCA should offer Tai Chi classes to nonmembers on a pay-as-you-go basis?"

Table 6.1 Example of a Focus Group Protocol

Phase	Specifics
Preparation	1. Make confirmation calls 24 to 48 hours ahead. 2. Purchase refreshments, tapes, and name tags. 3. Check tape recorder and batteries.
Set-up	1. Arrive 30 minutes ahead of scheduled start time to set up. 2. Bring tape recorder, 14 name tags, 14 copies of consent forms, background questionnaires, and any other materials.
Welcoming	1. Introduce yourselves as participants come in. 2. Make light conversation, especially if people do not know each other. 3. Allow 15 to 20 minutes for settling in and refreshments. 4. Give everyone a name tag (real names or pseudonyms).
Beginning the session (everyone is seated)	1. Facilitator makes formal introductions, explains the general purpose of the project, his or her role, and that of the recorder. 2. Facilitator hands out consent forms for participation and audiotaping. 3. Recorder makes a seating plan. Turn on tape recorder with permission.
Setting the ground rules	1. Facilitator establishes the ground rules, such as the following: • We request that you speak one at a time so we don't miss anything. • There are no right or wrong answers. All comments are valuable. • It's okay to disagree—everyone has different opinions.
Following the script	1. Facilitator begins with the icebreaker question, followed by transitional questions, key questions, and summary questions. 2. For each question on the script, the recorder notes the name of every speaker and the beginning of his or her comment. For instance, after question 1 was posed, John spoke first: "Well, I think that..."Judy broke in: "I disagree, transportation is a concern...." 3. Facilitator closely monitors the time and coverage of the script.
Administering background form (optional)	1. Facilitator hands out a form and pen to each person, saying, "Now take a few minutes to complete the checklist to give us a general description of the people taking part in the discussion session.
Closing and getting follow-up consent	1. Facilitator summarizes main points of the discussion and asks whether people have anything to add. 2. Facilitator explains follow-up for verification and hands out consent form for telephone follow-up. 3. Facilitator thanks participants and perhaps give them certificates or gifts.

Table 6.2 Focus Group Scripts for Evaluating the Corporate Fitness Class and Exercise Equipment

Samples	Continuing participants	Dropouts	Abstainers
Purpose of evaluation project	To explore why they joined the aerobics class and continue to participate, and whether they also use the equipment.	To explore why they dropped out of the aerobics class, and whether they use the equipment.	To explore why they did not sign up for the class, and whether they use the on-site exercise equipment.
Icebreaker Round-robin questions, everyone answers	Let's go around the table; tell us how long you've been attending the aerobics class.	Let's go around the table; tell us how long you attended the aerobics class.	Let's go around the table; do you belong to any exercise programs or clubs? Do you work out? Describe.
Introductory question To introduce the topic	How did you hear about the aerobics class? You've seen the equipment in the studio. Have you tried it? What specifically?	How did you hear about the aerobics class? You've seen the equipment in the studio. Have you tried it? What specifically?	Do you know about the exercise room on the first floor? What do we offer in our exercise studio?
Transition question To move the conversation to key questions	What prompted you to join the aerobics class? Do you know anyone the class?	What prompted you to join the aerobics class? Did you know anyone in the class?	Why didn't you try the class? Have you tried the exercise equipment? What specifically?
Key questions In-depth examination	What keeps you coming back? Is there anything you would like changed? Prompts—time, music, etc. Other types of classes or equipment you would like?	Why did you discontinue? Is there anything we could do to get you to return? Other types of classes or equipment you would like?	Is there anything we could change about the aerobics class to get you to join? Would you be interested in other types of classes? Other exercise equipment?
Summary question	These are the main points raised today.... Do you agree? Is there anything you'd like to add?	These are the main points raised today.... Do you agree? Is there anything you'd like to add?	These are the main points raised today.... Do you agree? Is there anything you'd like to add?

• *Summary* or *closure questions* wrap up the discussion and provide the opportunity for participants to clarify their positions or add comments. For instance, "A great deal of useful information was brought out today. I think the main points that you felt strongly about were . . . . Do you agree that these were the main points? Is there anything anyone would like to add?"

Another example of focus group scripts is shown in table 6.2 for evaluating the corporate fitness program scenario. Note that different scripts are used for conducting separate groups with continuing participants, dropouts, and abstainers, because the purpose of the evaluation project is different with each group.

Several tips to keep in mind when developing focus group scripts include the following:

• Limit the number of dichotomous questions, which participants can answer yes or no.

• Use open-ended questions to promote discussion.

• Have prompts ready to get people to elaborate or provide detailed remarks.

• Keep the number of questions to a minimum so you discuss all pertinent issues. A total of five or six questions can usually generate an hour-long discussion! Questions may need prompts or probing statements to get people talking.

In the best possible scenario, focus groups basically run themselves, the discussion naturally flows and evolves, and everyone contributes to the discussion. The facilitator may find that the remaining questions in the script have already been addressed as the discussion unfolds. He or she may simply need to tie things together in the summary or closing section.

Step 6 Develop Consent Forms

Refer to worksheets 6.6 through 6.8 for sample consent forms specifically designed for focus group projects. I prefer the less technical term discussion group (over focus group) when recruiting or speaking to participants. Explain and administer the first two forms—consent for group discussions (worksheet 6.6) and consent for audiotaping

Worksheet 6.6
Consent Form for Group Discussions

I understand that I am agreeing to take part in a 90-minute discussion with 5 to 10 other people to explore the possibility of developing a new program and to help plan this new program. I may choose when, and if, to make comments during the discussion. At the end of the session, I will complete a short checklist that should take about 10 minutes. It is my choice whether to complete this checklist.

My participation is totally voluntary and in no way will affect the services I now receive or may receive in the future. You will give everyone pseudonyms (false names) at the beginning to protect confidentiality. You will put no names on the checklist. You will summarize the information from both the discussion and the checklists across this group, and other discussion groups, to provide viewpoints and a general description of the men and women taking part.

Consent Form

You have explained the purpose of this project to my satisfaction, and I have had the opportunity to ask questions. I will receive a copy of this consent form. If I have any questions or concerns arising from my participation, I should feel free to contact _____.

Participant's name (please print) _____

Participant's signature _____ Date _____

Worksheet 6.7
Consent Form for Audiotaping

We need the permission of all participants to audiotape the discussion session. The reason for audiotaping is so we do not miss the valuable comments people make. The tapes allow us to go back and analyze the data more completely. We may site specific comments in the reports, but will identify no individuals. We will keep the tapes secure and destroy them following analysis. Do you have any questions?

- -

Consent Form

You have explained the reasons for audiotaping the discussion session to my satisfaction. I understand that everyone in the group has to agree before audiotaping will take place. By signing below, I am consenting to the audiotaping.

Participant's name (please print) _____

Participant's signature _____ Date _____

(worksheet 6.7)—at the start of the session. Explain and administer the third form—consent for follow-up verification (worksheet 6.8)—at the end of the session. Refer to the protocol in table 6.1.

Step 7 Advertise and Recruit

Once you have developed your protocol, script, and consent forms and tentatively scheduled your personnel, rooms, and equipment, you are ready to proceed with recruitment.

When we recruit for focus groups, we use separate sign-up sheets for each prebooked date and time period. As individuals sign up (name and phone number), we hand them an appointment card (which specifies the date, time, and location) as well as a letter of information about the project and who to call for further information or cancellation. We also have a general sign-up sheet for interested volunteers who cannot make any prescheduled sessions.

Provide participants with a reminder, confirmation phone call 24 to 48 hours before the scheduled session. If your participants are over age 40, remind them to bring their reading glasses. Because people inevitably cancel at the last minute, it is a good idea to book up to 14 people for each

session. Another reason you will need their phone numbers is to reschedule if fewer than six people sign up for a session.

Step 8 Prepare for Session

Following recruitment, there should be a list of things to do to get ready for each session. Some things you'll want to take care of before the session include the following:

1. Confirm the session times with the facilitator and volunteers 24 to 48 hours before the event.
2. Confirm that the room is reserved.
3. Prepare adequate copies of needed consent forms, blank name tags, and pencils.
4. Prepare hat with pseudonyms (if needed).
5. Have session script printed.
6. Check tape recorder, batteries, and tapes.
7. Purchase refreshments, cups, napkins, and so on for participants.

On the day of the session, the facilitator and recorder should arrive about 30 minutes ahead of participants to set up. Follow the protocol as in table 6.1.

Step 9 Conduct Session

At the beginning of the discussion session (once everyone is seated), the recorder makes a detailed seating plan, similar to the one in figure 6.2, and records the name of each person around the table (including the facilitator and the recorder).

During the session, the recorder takes notes concerning who speaks the most or least, non-verbal gestures, such as head nodding at specific points in the discussion, whether participants knew one another and addressed their remarks to certain people, areas of agreement or disagreement, and so on. As noted in the sample protocol (table 6.1), as the facilitator poses each question, the recorder should make a note of each speaker, in turn, and the opening part of each person's remarks. This will make it easier to match your field notes with who is speaking when you later listen to the tapes.

Worksheet 6.8
Consent Form for Follow-Up Verification

Thank you for taking part in the discussion group today. The information provided will assist (name of organization) in planning this new program (or improving a current program). When we analyze the data, we will look for themes or issues arising from each group and then summarize the findings across groups.

To ensure that we have accurately captured the primary issues that emerged from each session, we would like to contact a few participants in each group two to four weeks from now. We will conduct a 15-minute follow-up by telephone to: (1) verify the findings, see if participants agree with the major points we felt emerged from the discussion; and (2) see whether participants have any further thoughts to add.

Giving your permission allows us to contact you by phone two to four weeks from now. If we randomly select your consent form, one of the facilitators you have met today will contact you. If you still agree at that time, we will set up a convenient time for the 15-minute conversation. We may not contact you at all, and we certainly would only contact you once. If you do not wish to participate or participation is inconvenient, no further calls will take place. We will keep these forms secure and destroy them once we have contacted you or we determine we have a sufficient number of respondents. We will not give out your name and number to anyone or use it for any purpose apart from this project. Do you have any questions?

Consent Form

You have explained the purpose of this follow-up to my satisfaction, and I have had the opportunity to ask questions. By signing below, I give my permission for one of the facilitators I have met today to call me at the number below to arrange a 15-minute follow-up by phone. I understand that I may not agree at that time to the interview. Should I decline, you will make no further contact and will destroy this form.

Printed name _____   Phone number _____

Signature _____   Date _____

Most convenient days to call ___ Mon   ___ Tues   ___ Wed   ___ Thur   ___ Fri

Best time to call ___ morning ___ afternoon ___ early evening

Field notes are your recorded observations and impressions, during and immediately following each focus group session. It is important to write down and complete your field notes soon after the session while your impressions are still fresh (and so you will not get confused by the next session). After both the facilitator and recorder have independently jotted down their field notes, they should get together and debrief.

Step 10 Debrief

The *debriefing* process is essentially a postsession examination by the facilitator and the recorder. The two observers discuss their impressions of the session itself and participant interactions. You can standardize the process by covering some key areas, such as "Did everyone contribute to the discussion? Did anyone stand out in terms of their experiences or opinions? What were the main areas of agreement or disagreement? Did people feel particularly strong or emotional about certain issues?" Either take detailed notes or tape record the debriefing.

Be certain to label each piece of information (tapes, seating charts, background questionnaires, consent forms, debriefing notes) according to the location, date, and time of the particular session, as well as the personnel who conducted the session. Remember, you will usually conduct at least two focus groups for each evaluation project. You do not want to get the information from different sessions confused.

Step 11 Revise Script and Proceed to Next Session

Immediately following the first session of a project, reexamine the protocol and script and make revisions, if necessary, before the next session. For instance, you may want to schedule an additional break. You may find that there were too many questions for the session duration, or, some questions may have generated yes or no responses and required additional prompts to get people talking. Some prompts work better than others. Make notes on the protocol and script itself in preparation for the next session.

Although it is okay to shorten the number of questions and add prompts, be sure you ask your most important questions again at the next session. You cannot compare the findings from different sessions unless you have collected basically

the same information in each. Repeat steps 8 through 10 with all remaining sessions.

Step 12 Analyze the Findings

Your seating plan, field notes, debriefing notes, and the tape-recorded discussion session constitute your data. You may also have administered a background questionnaire at the end of the session.

Analyze the data after the first two sessions—these results will determine whether you need to conduct further sessions. You will also need to verify your primary findings by contacting a random sample of participants from each group by telephone. Two or three people from each session will suffice. Recall that you must obtain permission for follow-up contact before participants leave their session (see worksheet 6.8). Chapter 7 shows you how to analyze and interpret focus group data.

Assessing Client Outcomes

Information from background questionnaires administered to all clients at the time of entry and individual attendance records are critical sources of information for outcome evaluation. If you do not routinely collect these two types of information, you will need to collect it for the sample of clients who participate in the outcome evaluation project. It is important to examine which clients improve the most! Background characteristics and attendance rates are essential in this regard.

You need to collect background information on clients only once, because most of this information will not change. A short follow-up questionnaire, however, is useful to examine whether there have been major disruptions in normal activity patterns and whether clients have started any new physical activities outside the class or program in question. For clients with chronic health problems, check whether there have been any changes in their symptoms. Worksheet 6.9 provides an example of a follow-up questionnaire.

You can also use worksheet 6.9 to obtain client impressions on the program and personal benefits. As discussed in chapter 5, however, simply asking clients whether they think they have improved as a result of participation (retrospective reports) is not highly credible. Clients may have trouble recalling what they were like before (memory bias)

Worksheet 6.9
Prototype Follow-Up Questionnaire

Name or ID _____ Date completed _____

It has now been about ____ month(s) since you began your exercise class and completed our background questionnaire. We hope you will take the time to answer a few questions, complete a few short scales, and give us feedback on the class. Remember, we will keep this information strictly confidential.

1. Since you joined this class, have any events **caused a major disruption in your normal patterns of activity** (such as an illness or injury to yourself or someone close, or a job change, etc.)? ___ no ___ yes (specify _____)

2. Have you noticed **any change** in your _____ (fill in name of condition: arthritis, diabetes, low-back pain, asthma, etc.) in terms of _____ (fill in pain, breathing difficulty, or other relevant symptoms)? ____ improvement _____ about the same _____ worse

3. Since joining this class, **have you started any other physical activities** (classes, sports, or exercising on your own) **outside the class?** ___ no ___ yes

If yes, please complete the following chart.

Type of activity	How often per week	Where (e.g., home, pool, fitness center)
_____	_____	_____
_____	_____	_____

4. To what extent is exercising currently **an important part of your regular routine?**
(Circle number.)   1   2   3   4   5

	Not at all important		Moderately important		Extremely important

5. How **physically exerting** do you find this class?

(Circle number.)   1   2   3   4   5

	Not at all exerting		Moderately exerting		Overly exerting

6. How do you **usually feel** after the class?

(Circle number.)   1   2   3   4   5

	Not at all tired		Pleasantly tired		Unpleasantly tired or wiped out

7. Is there *anything* about this class you would like to see **changed** (for example, scheduling, location, music, level of exercise)? ____no ____ yes (please specify _____)

8. Finally, what have you **personally gained from this class**; what keeps you coming back?
_____
_____

Thank you for taking the time to complete this questionnaire. Your instructor may also ask you to complete some additional short forms. If so, they will be attached to this package. Please tell your instructor if you found any questions unclear. **Return the package according to your program leader's instructions.**

or may be trying to say positive things to please their instructor. For outcome evaluation, you need to do pre- and postassessments for each primary outcome measure.

Chapter 5 described an array of tools for outcome evaluation. Some tools, such as fitness assessments, you may routinely use in your program for initial screening and developing individualized exercise prescriptions. For outcome evaluation, conduct such appraisals consistently across clients, and reassess clients to determine whether fitness parameters (body mass index, aerobic capacity, strength, etc.) change. The same holds true for functional performance measures (examples in table 5.2) and self-report measures, such as self-efficacy and health status or well-being (examples in table 5.3). This section addresses when to administer such measures for outcome evaluation and how to obtain an adequate sample size.

Timing Considerations

Once you have selected and pilot tested your outcome measures, decide when to conduct pre- and postassessments. Conduct preassessments at *baseline* or *program entry*, that is, *before* clients have started the class or exercise regimen. It is *not* suitable to include ongoing participants, because they may have already improved. Timing of postassessments depends on several factors: the nature and length of the intervention, frequency of participation, and the baseline fitness level of participants.

The exercise literature in your area may be useful in making this determination. For instance, programs typically assess change following 12 weeks of participation at a frequency of three times a week for aerobic training regimens. For other types of exercise interventions and outcomes, however, a 12-week period may not be appropriate. For instance, we conducted our follow-up assessments to assess extent of recovery of injured workers after only three weeks, because this is when clients were typically discharged from these rehabilitation clinics (Williams and Myers 1998a).

Health and well-being outcome measures may show a different course of change than fitness outcomes. For instance, King et al. (1997) found that for people with moderate sleep complaints, sleep quality improved after 16 weeks (but not after only 8 weeks) of moderate intensity exercise. We found scores on the Vitality Plus Scale (see figure 5.2) improved with different types of exercise participation, but the course of improvement depended on the duration in the program and attendance rate (Myers et al. in press). If there are no relevant guidelines, you may have to use your best guesses based on experience and observation (how long do you think it takes for your clients to show improvements?), or you need to conduct several measures to determine *incremental change,* such as 4-week, 8-week, or 16-week comparisons. Keep in mind frequency of participation. Change should occur faster if clients are participating several times versus once a week. For some client groups, such as frail seniors or people with chronic illness, *maintenance* may be the desired outcome rather than improvement.

Sampling Considerations

As recommended in table 5.4, you should sample at least 30 people for an outcome evaluation (Mertens 1998). If you have a large client base of about 100 or 200 people, you may wish to select a smaller sample (of at least 30) for your outcome study, particularly if you have several measures. Keep in mind that the sample should be as representative as possible of your clientele. For instance, if your clientele includes men and women or people of different ages or fitness levels, you should select a sample that includes these characteristics.

Most likely, you will have smaller numbers of clients to work with. Let's say, for instance, that you keep class size to a maximum of 10 people.

Session 1 (10 clients)	Session 2 (10 clients)	Session 3 (10 clients)
Week 1 .... Week 12	Week 1 .... Week 12	Week 1 .... Week 12
Pretest .... Posttest	Pretest .... Posttest	Pretest .... Posttest

Figure 6.3 Staggered approach to data collection for outcome evaluation.

If you run multiple sections of a given class, you could gather information concurrently (at the same time) on three classes to achieve your desired sample size (3 × 10 = 30). If there were only 8 people in each section, you would need to combine four classes (4 × 8 = 32), and so on.

On the other hand, if you run classes sequentially (e.g., one session every 12 weeks), you will need to use a staggered approach to achieve your desired sample size, as in figure 6.3.

For the example in figure 6.3, it would take 9 months (or 36 weeks) to collect pre- and postdata on 30 clients by combining three consecutive cohorts. In contrast, if you run at least three sections of a given class (e.g., Tai Chi, aerobics, or weight training) concurrently, then you could collect pre- and postdata on 30 clients in only 12 weeks (assuming you conducted postassessments after three months of participation).

Sequential Approach

Finally, consider whether you want to include a comparison group in your outcome study to determine the relative effectiveness of one program over another. For instance, chapter 4 described our outcome evaluation of the FFLTC program, in which we compared a more challenging exercise class for nursing home residents with a less challenging, seated program. The former group showed substantial improvement on several measures (mobility, balance, strength, flexibility), but the latter group deteriorated on several measures over the same four-month period (Lazowski et al. in press).

It is highly unlikely that the recreation director in scenario 6 would be able to conduct such an elaborate outcome evaluation. It is more likely that she would choose only a few simple published measures, such as the TUG mobility test, compare her class participants before and after participation (say a four-month interval based on the Lazowski et al. (in press) findings, and use a simple formula (which I will describe in chapter 7) to calculate how many clients in her class improved. As discussed in chapter 4, programs should take a simple and sequential approach to examining client outcomes. First, examine whether clients in the program under evaluation change at all, how much, and over what period. Then, compare whether one program or exercise regimen is more beneficial than another.

Summary

This chapter addresses the most important types of information programs should collect for process evaluation and outcome evaluation, respectively. All programs should be able to profile their new (and existing) clientele and use the information to describe their clientele, to determine whether their client profile changes over time, and to identify characteristics of frequent users and dropouts. By knowing more about your dropouts, you can develop strategies to enhance adherence and address program barriers that are amenable to change.

Tracking participation rates is also something programs should do routinely. Although you can easily calculate aggregate or average usage rates from individual attendance records, the reverse is not true. This chapter also discussed assessing absentees and dropouts using a standard telephone protocol for contacting absent clients. Such procedures have been shown to reduce attrition and provide valuable evaluation information.

Focus groups may be the most useful strategy for obtaining in-depth feedback from potential consumers (for needs assessment and formative evaluation) and from current or former clients (for process evaluation). The step-by-step guidelines in this chapter are similar to what training workshops typically cover and should be sufficient to get you started. Your skills and comfort level will increase as you gain experience planning and conducting focus groups.

This chapter also addressed client-outcome measurement. Use a follow-up questionnaire to examine whether health conditions or lifestyle practices have changed over the intervening period. It is particularly important to determine whether people have joined other fitness facilities or started exercising on their own (outside the class or facility in question). However, be wary of relying on retrospective reports, because such information by itself will not be seen as highly credible. Assess clients before and after participation to determine change on the key measures of interest.

Now that we have gone through how to collect evaluation information, you need to know what to do with the information collected. Chapter 7 shows you how to manage, score, analyze, and interpret the information and how to report evaluation findings and recommendations.

Interpreting and Using Evaluation Information

Once you have collected your data, there are a few remaining tasks. First, you need to manage the information you've collected. Second, you need to analyze this information. Third, you need to interpret and use your evaluation findings. In addition, you may need, or want, to present the evaluation findings to other stakeholders. This chapter provides guidelines and suggestions for managing, analyzing, interpreting, using, and presenting evaluation findings.

Managing Information

Exercise programs vary widely regarding whether they use manual or computer-based (electronic or automated) information management. The larger the client base and the greater the number of programs or services provided, the more likely your agency or facility is already using computer spreadsheets to keep track of payrolls, equipment purchases and repair costs, client payments, and mailing lists. Even large facilities, however, may still store some types of client information—registration forms, medical histories, fitness appraisals, client-satisfaction surveys—manually in file folders.

Let's take a simple example, client-satisfaction surveys, to illustrate challenges in data management. Anonymous client-satisfaction surveys are commonly stored in separate files by program and by year (or time) of the survey. Table 3.2 (p. 36) illustrated a summary of a single client-satisfaction survey. You could manually produce such

a summary by going through all 100 questionnaires and recording each response to each of the 11 questions. You could use a hand calculator to calculate totals. Let's say you wanted to compare the findings across five years of such surveys. Again, you could manually score each batch and work with the annual summary sheets. You could do the same if you wanted to compare satisfaction ratings for a given year across classes.

However, it would be much easier if all this information was contained in a computer database. You only need to enter the information once, then the computer does the work for you—calculating totals for each survey question, comparing totals from year to year (or class to class), and producing tables or graphs to display the results. Computers eliminate having to find storage space for numerous boxes of surveys, and you are less likely to lose computer files than paper files that may be several years old!

As the amount of information increases, so does the necessity for computer-based data management. Look at the prototype background questionnaire (worksheet 6.4, p. 92). If you collected all this information for every new client, it would soon become a logistic nightmare to interpret without computer assistance. Remember you will want to take advantage of this information to compare your client profile over time and to compare profiles of adherers and dropouts. Computer databases are also essential if you want to link different sources of information, such as client outcomes, characteristics, and attendance rates.

The good news is that computer hardware and software is inexpensive and easy to use. Whether you already have a computer at your facility, or plan to purchase one, here is what you will need for evaluation purposes. The most important feature is that the computer has the capacity or memory to store and manage large quantities of information (at least 8 megs of RAM; 16 megs is preferable).

You will need software packages (some may come with the computer) for the following: word processing, data management, data analyses, and data graphing. There is an array of software on the market to choose from. Word processing packages, such as Microsoft Word or WordPerfect, are useful for typing memos and reports. Although these packages can create tables, they are not good for manipulating numbers. You need additional software for data management, processing, and graphical display. Some spreadsheet programs are useful for financial accounting (e.g., Lotus) but may not contain the analytical (statistical) tools needed for evaluation. The software must be able to compute simple descriptive statistics, such as means and frequencies; comparative statistics, such as cross tabulations; and work with formulas (for calculating membership growth, attrition, and client change). I will explain and illustrate these simple statistics later in this chapter.

Some software packages, such as SPSS (Statistical Package for Social Sciences), are specifically designed to analyze numeric data. Other soft-

ware, such as NUD*IST (Non-Numerical Unstructured Data Indexing Searching and Theorizing), is specifically designed for working with qualitative data. Researchers use such software programs, and they are more elaborate than most programs need for evaluation purposes. Furthermore, SPSS and NUD*IST have limited built-in graphical capabilities. You will likely need to use another program, such as PowerPoint or Excel, to visually display and present your evaluation findings.

Thus, in addition to a word processor, you need software for data entry and management, manipulation or analysis, and graphing. Microsoft Excel is an example of a data software package that is user-friendly for data processing. Excel provides an adequate range of statistical tools and allows you to create your own formulas for analysis. There are over 100 charting options for displaying your results.

Data Coding and Entry

You will need to become familiar with the conventions and limitations for data entry and manipulation associated with the software package you choose. Don't be confused by the different terminology used by different software programs. *Databases* may be called workbooks (e.g., in Excel) or notebooks (e.g., in Corel Quattro). *Data files*, which make up a database, may be called spreadsheets, worksheets, or pages. Most people are familiar with the term *spreadsheet* for financial reporting or keeping track of home mortgage interest payments. In this chapter, we use the terms databases and data files (or spreadsheets); data files and spreadsheets are interchangeable terms.

Each software program has rules governing the amount and format of information that you can put into each data file or spreadsheet. Most programs designed for data management can handle well over 200 columns and thousands of rows of information (e.g., Corel Quattro can handle over 8,000; Excel can handle over 16,000) for each spreadsheet. I am going to show you some spreadsheets, but these examples are limited by how much information I can put on a standard page. An actual spreadsheet filled to capacity displayed on a single sheet of paper could stretch the length of several cars and the height of an office tower!

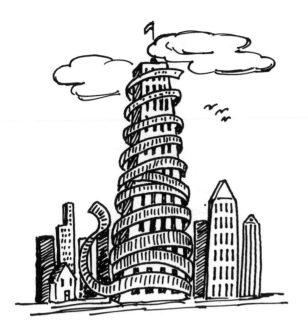

Although a single spreadsheet or data file can hold an incredible amount of information, it is easier for novices to work with the information if you create separate data files for each type of information. For your evaluation database, I recommend that you create separate data files for

- client-background information,
- attendance records for each program,
- fitness assessment information,
- each inventory or scale you administer,
- each client-satisfaction survey, and
- information from structured telephone interviews with absent clients.

Separate files are easier to manage and analyze. You can easily bring in or link information from various files when needed.

Data files consist of *columns* and *rows*. Rows represent people. Each row contains information on only one client. Columns represent variables. The intersection of a row and column is called a *cell*. Each cell contains a specific piece of information (e.g., a person's age). You will need to develop a codebook for each data file to guide you in data entry and interpretation. The next sections show you illustrations of codebooks and spreadsheets.

Codebooks

As the term implies, a *codebook* is your manual or guide for data entry. Develop a codebook for each

data file. The codebook tells you where each piece of information is located, describes what each piece of information represents (by variable name or label), and specifies what the values or numbers in each cell mean (by descriptors).

I have developed two sample codebooks for illustration. The first codebook (see worksheet 7.1) is for the prototype background questionnaire in worksheet 6.4 (p. 92). Referring to this background questionnaire, you will see that there are 32 questions numbered sequentially under four parts (A, demographic; B, health; C, current activities; and D, program-related questions). I have chosen to label the first two columns ID number and Completion date. The subsequent columns are labeled by part and question number (A1, A2, etc.). The variable names describe the type of information in each column. The descriptors denote the values for each variable entered into the data file or spreadsheet. For example, for gender, I chose 1 = Male and 2 = Female. Various software programs use different conventions to denote missing values or information. Excel uses blanks for missing information as I have done in this sample codebook.

I have provided illustrations for coding about a third of this questionnaire (you will need to complete the codebook). As you can see, coding forced-choice questions, such as gender or employment category, is straightforward. Coding open-ended questions or options, such as other categories, however, is more difficult. The codebook provides some examples, for instance question 10 (when respondents list "other" health problems), question 11 (listing of medications), question 15 (how they spend their leisure time), and question 27 (how they heard about the program). Under the qualitative data analysis section later in this chapter, I describe how to do a content analysis for data such as written responses to open-ended questions.

The second example of a codebook is for class attendance data (see worksheet 7.2). You could use a generic codebook, as shown in the example, for all your classes or programs, or create individual codebooks for each class or class type (e.g., daily classes or weekly sessions). In any case, keep separate data files for each class (each with a unique *file name*, such as Aerobic Attendance or Tai Chi Attendance). The example in worksheet 7.2 contains separate columns for days offered and for time slots. You may wish to include other

Worksheet 7.1
Sample Codebook for Prototype Background Questionnaire

Column	Variable label	Descriptors
ID #	Client ID number	Month/day/year/order of entry (e.g., two clients join on 1/1/98: the first is allocated 1/1/98/1, the second is allocated 1/1/98/2)
Date	Completion date	Month/day/year
A1	Gender	1 = Male 2 = Female Blank = Missing data
A2	Birth date	Month/day/year
A3	Education	1 = Did not complete high school 2 = Completed high school 3 = Completed college Blank = Missing data
A4	Employment	1 = Full time 2 = Part time 3 = Self-employed 4 = Between jobs 5 = Homemaker or caretaker 6 = Student 7 = Semiretired 8 = Fully retired Blank = Missing or ambiguous (checked more than one category)
B6	Health state	1 = Excellent 2 = Good 3 = Fair 4 = Poor Blank = Missing
B10	Total health problems	Possible range 0 to 20

B10a	Heart trouble	0 = No (not checked)
B10b	COPD	1 = Yes (checked)
B10c	Diabetes	Blank = Missing
B10d	Osteoporosis	
B10e	Arthritis	
B10f	Blood pressure	
B10g	Cholesterol	
B10h	Overweight	
B10i	Back	
B10j	Foot	
B10k	Allergies	
B10l	Hearing	
B10m	Vision	
B10n	Cancer	
B10o	Epilepsy	
B10p	Parkinson's	
B10q	Other	
B10r	Other	
B11	Number of medications	0 = No 1 = Yes (checked or one listed) n = Number of medications listed Blank = Missing
B11a	Heart med	0 = Not listed
B11b	Pain med	1 = Listed
B11c	BP med	Blank = Missing (said yes to B11)
B11d	Insulin	
B11e		
B11f		
B11g		
B13	Limitation	0 = No 1 = Yes, temporary 2 = Yes, long-term Blank = Missing
C14	Leisure hours Hours on a given weekday	0 to ..... Number of hours specified Blank = Missing

continued

Column	Variable label	Descriptors
C15a1 C15a2 C15a3 C15a4 C15a5 C15a6	Your time What do you usually do in leisure time? (allows up to six separate responses per person)	1 = Reading 2 = Watching TV 3 = Sports 4 = 5= 6 = Blank = Missing
C15b1 C15b2 C15b3 C15b4 C15b5 C15b6	People time What do you usually do in leisure time with others?	1= 2 = 3 = 4 = 5 = 6 = Blank = Missing
C18	Importance Importance of exercise or sport as part of routine	1 = Not at all important 2 = 3 = Moderately important 4 = 5 = Extremely important Blank = Missing
D27	Hear about	1 = Word of mouth, unspecified 2 = Word of mouth, relative 3 = Word of mouth, friend 4 = Newspaper 5 = Radio 6 = Poster 7 = 8 = Blank = Missing

types of information, such as the gender and age of each instructor, class location, and so on.

Spreadsheets

I created two hypothetical spreadsheets for illustration purposes using a word processor table option. In reality, entering data into a computer data spreadsheet is much easier, because you do not have to worry about page size and column widths. You just need to put your cursor in the right place and enter the information into each cell. You will enter most data manually unless you have the capabilities to scan information directly into the computer. Software programs usually have checks to catch human errors—mistakes in manual data entry. For instance, say your valid codes for a variable were

Worksheet 7.2
Sample Codebook for Class Attendance Data Entry

Filename	Column	Variable label	Descriptors
Attendance, aerobics Attendance, aquafit Attendance, Tai Chi Attendance, weight Attendance,			
	A	Type	1 = High impact 2 = Low impact 3 = 4 = 5 = 6 =
	B1 to B7 B1 = Mon B2 = Tues B3 = Wed B4 = Thur B5 = Fri B6 = Sat B7 = Sun	Days Days offered	0 = Not offered 1 = Offered
	C1 to C7 C1 = Before 9 A.M. C2 = 9 A.M. to noon C3 = Noon to 1 P.M. C4 = 1 P.M. to 4 P.M. C5 = 4 P.M. to 6 P.M. C6 = 6 P.M. to 9 P.M. C7 = After 9 P.M.	Time Time slot	0 = Not offered 1 = Offered
	ID #	Participant ID	Month/day/year/ order of entry (e.g., two clients join on 1/1/98 and are assigned 1/1/98/1 and 1/1/98/2, respectively)

continued

Filename	Column	Variable label	Descriptors
	S1 to S.... (or M1 = 1st Mon, W1 = 1st Wed, etc.	Session #	Record attendance for each registered participant for each consecutive session 1 = Present 2 = Absent Blank = Did not record X = Session cancelled

0 and 1. If you entered a 2 or 5 by mistake, the computer would tell you that this is an invalid entry.

The first example spreadsheet (worksheet 7.3) shows the class attendance pattern of 15 participants over a five-week period. Each data file requires a name to keep it distinct from other class attendance files. I have chosen to label the columns S1, S2, S3, and so on, to represent each session. As in the worksheet 7.2, the unique client ID number represents month/day/year/order of entry into the club or facility. The values in the cells represent whether each person was present (1) or absent (0) the day of the session. I chose an X to denote when a session was canceled. In your spreadsheet, you could have many more rows for additional participants and a vast number of columns for subsequent sessions.

The second example spreadsheet (worksheet 7.4) is for Vitality Plus Scale (VPS) scores at baseline and follow-up. I show a description of this 10-item measure, as well as directions for administering and scoring, in figure 5.2 (p. 78).

I chose to label each item from a1 to j1 at baseline (and from a2 to j2 at follow-up) as shown in the spreadsheet columns. This allows me to distinguish each item (a = fall asleep quickly, b = sleep well, down to j = feel good). Each item and time of administration must have a separate code. You want to be able to compare the total scores for the scale at time 1 and time 2. You may also want to examine change on particular items, such as energy or sleep on the VPS. Scores for this scale on each item can range from 1 to 5 (the values inserted into each cell for each person). Separate

variables (T1 and T2) represent the total VPS scores for each person at baseline and follow-up, respectively.

Note that the last row (15) contains blank cells; this means that this person did not complete the inventory. According to the scale developers' instructions (see figure 5.2, p. 78), a total score could not be computed for this client at baseline, because there was too much missing data (only 3 of the 10 items were answered). A total score could be computed at follow-up, however, by taking the average for the 8 items answered ($32 \div 8 = 4$), and inserting this value for the missing items. We will work further with this example in the next section on analysis.

Analyzing Quantitative Data

Much of your evaluation data will be quantitative or numerical, such as forced-choice responses, ratings on background questionnaires or client-satisfaction surveys, attendance rates, and scores on fitness appraisals, performance, or self-report inventories.

Once you have entered the data into a computer data file, the computer's analytical or statistical tools can help you make sense of the data. As previously mentioned, there are three types of statistical procedures you will need to use for quantitative evaluation information: descriptive, comparative, and formulas. This section describes each procedure, when to use it, and how to interpret the resulting information.

Worksheet 7.3
Sample Spreadsheet for Class Attendance

		Week 1			Week 2				Week 3			Week 4		Week 5		
	ID #	S1	S2	S3	S4	S5	S6	S7	S8	S9	S10	S11	S12	S13	S14	S15
1	5/6/96/1	1	1	X	1	0	1	1	1	1	1	0	0	1	X	1
2	2/7/97/1	1	1	X	1	1	1	1	1	1	1	1	1	1	X	1
3	1/5/98/2	1	0	X	0	0	0	0	0	0	0	0	0	0	X	0
4	4/10/97/1	1	1	X	1	1	1	1	1	0	1	1	0	1	X	0
5	3/5/98/3	1	0	X	0	1	0	0	0	0	0	0	0	0	X	0
6	1/5/98/1	1	1	X	1	1	0	1	1	0	1	1	0	1	X	0
7	10/5/97/1	1	1	X	1	1	1	1	1	0	1	1	1	1	X	1
8	4/30/98/1	1	1	X	1	1	0	1	1	0	1	1	0	1	X	0
9	3/27/97/1	1	1	X	1	1	1	1	0	0	0	0	0	0	X	0
10	2/14/96/2	1	1	X	1	1	0	1	1	0	1	1	0	1	X	0
11	3/28/98/1	1	1	X	1	1	0	1	1	1	1	1	0	0	X	1
12	5/31/97/1	1	0	X	1	0	1	0	1	0	1	0	1	0	X	0
13	9/22/97/1	1	1	X	1	1	1	1	1	0	1	0	1	1	X	1
14	10/20/96/1	1	1	X	1	0	0	0	0	0	0	1	0	0	X	0
15	08/15/97/2	1	1	X	1	0	0	0	0	1	1	1	1	1	X	1

Worksheet 7.4
Sample Spreadsheet for Vitality Plus Scale (VPS) Scores at Baseline and Follow-Up

ID #	a1	b1	c1	d1	e1	f1	g1	h1	i1	j1	T1	a2	b2	c2	d2	e2	f2	g2	h2	i2	j2	T2
1 1/5/98/1	1	2	2	5	4	4	2	4	2	3	**29**	5	4	5	5	5	4	5	4	4	5	**46**
2 1/5/98/2	5	5	5	5	5	5	5	5	5	5	**50**	5	5	5	5	5	5	5	5	5	5	**50**
3 1/6/98/1	3	4	4	2	2	3	2	5	3	3	**31**	3	4	5	4	4	4	4	5	4	4	**41**
4 1/7/98/1	4	4	4	5	5	5	5	5	5	5	**47**	5	4	4	5	5	5	5	5	5	5	**48**
5 1/9/98/1	2	2	2	2	4	4	5	4	4	4	**33**	4	4	4	3	4	4	5	5	5	5	**43**
6 1/12/98/1	4	4	4	4	4	4	4	4	4	4	**40**	3	4	4	4	4	4	4	5	4	4	**40**
7 1/14/98/1	1	1	1	5	5	3	1	4	2	3	**26**	3	3	4	5	5	4	4	4	4	4	**40**
8 1/16/98/1	3	3	3	3	3	3	4	5	4	4	**35**	3	4	4	3	5	5	4	5	5	5	**43**
9 1/16/98/2	5	5	5	5	5	4	5	4	5	5	**48**	5	5	5	5	5	4	5	4	5	5	**48**
10 1/16/98/3	2	3	3	5	5	5	3	5	5	4	**40**	4	5	5	5	5	5	5	5	5	5	**49**
11 1/19/98/1	4	4	4	5	5	5	5	5	5	5	**47**	4	5	4	5	5	5	5	5	5	5	**48**
12 1/23/98/1	5	5	5	5	5	5	5	5	5	5	**50**	5	5	5	5	5	5	5	5	5	5	**50**
13 1/24/98/1	3	2	2	5	4	3	3	4	3	3	**32**	4	4	4	5	4	4	4	4	4	4	**41**
14 1/27/98/1	1	1	1	2	1	1	1	2	2	1	**13**	4	3	3	4	4	4	4	4	5	2	**37**
15 1/31/98/1	3	4	5								—	4	5	5	3	4	4	3	4	5		**40**

Descriptive Analyses

Descriptive analyses help you make sense of large volumes of information. For instance, the prototype background questionnaire (worksheet 6.4) contains 32 questions. If you administered this questionnaire to only 50 clients, you would still have 1,600 pieces of information to deal with. You want to summarize information on age, gender, education, and so on across individuals to obtain an overall picture, profile, or description of your clientele. There are basically two types of descriptive statistics—measures of central tendency and measures of frequency.

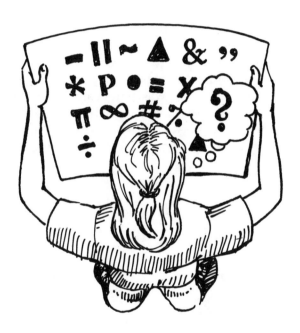

Measures of Central Tendency

Measures of central tendency describe the location and distribution of *continuous variables*. Age reported in years (e.g., 26 or 43) is an example of a continuous variable. For any group (a sample, a class, or an entire facility), you can compute the average age (mean), midpoint of the distribution (median), most common or frequently reported age (mode), minimum and maximum age (range), and variability around the mean (standard deviation). Most programs rely primarily on means and ranges for descriptive purposes.

In addition to age, other examples of continuous variables from the background questionnaire (worksheet 6.4) include total number of health problems (as determined from question 10); num-

ber of medications (question 11); perceived importance of exercising (from the 1 to 5 rating scale, question 18); activity level (number of days per week, question 22); and confidence (question 31). Number of sessions attended; fitness appraisal scores (aerobic capacity, weight, BMI, strength scores, etc.); scores on performance measures, such as walk speed; and scores on psychological inventories, such as the ABC and VPS scales shown in figures 5.1 and 5.2, are also continuous variables.

Measures of Frequency

You must describe categorical information, on the other hand, in terms of frequencies, percentages, ranks, or percentiles. Gender is an example of a categorical variable (male or female). You can also collect age information categorically, for instance, if you ask people to check whether they are in their 20s, 30s, 40s, and so on. In this case, you could *not* compute an average or mean age. You can, however, look at the frequency distribution to determine how many clients are in each age category (number and percentage). It is important to note that you can convert continuous information into categorical information, but not vice versa. For instance, you could group everyone in his or her 20s together, but knowing someone is in his 20s cannot tell you whether he is 20 or 25.

Other examples of categorical information from the background questionnaire in worksheet 6.4 include all questions with yes or no response formats, employment category, financial situation, perceived health, and so on. Demographic and other survey questions often use a categorical response format (checklist) to make it easier for respondents.

Comparative Analyses

Always start with descriptive statistics to get an overview of your data. By performing descriptive statistics for all the background information obtained from the prototype questionnaire, you are able to report the number of males and females, the average age, and many other characteristics of your sample. However, descriptive statistics alone cannot tell you whether your female clients are older than your male clients, which clients are more physically active, and so on. You need to do further, comparative, analyses of your descriptive data to answer such questions. *Comparative* analyses, as the term implies, allows you to compare different types of information, such as gender by age distributions.

There are many types of comparative analyses or statistical procedures. The ones you are most likely to use are

- cross tabulations (or chi-squares) to compare frequency data,
- *t*-tests to compare continuous variables, and
- correlations to compare continuous variables.

Let's look at some examples.

Let's say you conducted a survey of your membership to determine whether people were in favor of building a pool and whether they were willing to pay additional dues for this purpose. You sent out 250 surveys to a random sample of 125 female and 125 male members, and 180 people (102 females and 78 males) returned the survey questionnaire. A total of 118 were in favor of the pool, and 62 were opposed. A total of 84 respondents supported additional dues to build the pool, and 96 were opposed. Let's say you wanted to

know whether there was a gender difference; were more females or males in favor of the pool?

Chi-Square Statistic

You can examine this question using the cross tabulation or the chi-square statistic to test whether the proportion of males and females in favor was significantly different. The top of figure 7.1 illustrates a computer printout for a chi-square analysis based on the above data. The bottom of figure 7.1 shows you how to calculate a chi-square using a hand calculator.

As the formula illustrates, the chi-square statistical test compares the observed and expected frequencies to see whether one group's preferences are significantly different from another group's preferences. If you calculated the chi-square by hand, you would need to look up the result (6.57) in a statistical table to determine whether the finding was significant. Most general introductory level statistics books (cf. Armitage and Berry 1987; Welkowitz, Ewen, and Cohen 1971) contain tables with the significance

	Count Row % Column %	In favor Yes 1	No 2	Total
Gender	Male 1	43 55.1 36.4	35 44.9 56.5	78
	Female 2	75 73.5 63.6	27 26.4 43.5	102
		118	62	180

Chi-square	Value	DF	Significance
Likelihood ratio	6.57	1	.05

Formula: $\text{Chi}^2 = \sum \dfrac{(fo - fe)^2}{fe}$

where fo = observed frequency
fe = expected frequency
$\sum$ = is taken over all the categories

$fe = \dfrac{\text{(row total) (column total)}}{N}$

example: $\dfrac{78 \times 118}{180} = 51.1$

df = (r − 1) (c − 1) where r = number of rows and c = number of columns

fo	fe	fo − fe	$(fo - fe)^2$	$\dfrac{(fo - fe)^2}{fe}$
43	51.1	− 8.1	65.6	1.28
35	26.9	8.1	65.6	2.44
75	66.9	8.1	65.6	0.98
27	35.1	− 8.1	65.6	1.87

$\text{Chi}^2 = 6.57$

Figure 7.1 A chi-square analysis showing a computer printout and a manual calculation.

levels of chi-square values, *t*-test values, and correlational values. Such books are likely to be available at your public library or local bookstore.

It is easier to let the computer do this calculation for you. You simply tell the computer you want to do a 2 × 2 cross tabulation or chi-square (depending on what your software calls it), comparing the following variables: gender (1 = male, 2 = female) and in favor (1 = yes, 2 = no). The software will perform the calculations and produce a printout using the variable labels you entered. Printouts contain row and column percentages, the resulting chi-square (or likelihood ratio) value, the degrees of freedom (df) and the significance level. All you have to know is how to interpret the significance level.

In this example, the significance level is .05 (it could also be portrayed as $p < .05$). This means that the probability (p) that your finding was due to chance is only five times out of 100. If your result was significant at the $p < .01$ level, or at the $p < .001$, you would have even more confidence that your finding was not due to chance. You should not interpret values greater than .05 (e.g., .25 or .10) as a significant difference.

Because the finding in this case was $p < .05$, you can confidently conclude that the females surveyed were significantly more in favor of building the pool than the males surveyed. Not surprisingly, another chi-square analysis indicated that those in favor of building the pool were also significantly more likely to be in favor of paying additional dues for this purpose (here the significance level was $p < .001$).

Table 7.1 illustrates other examples of when the chi-square test would be appropriate to compare your data. For instance, you may want to compare the profile of adherers and dropouts based on information contained in the background questionnaire (administered when each client entered the fitness facility or exercise program).

As shown in table 7.1, you could use the chi-square test to compare whether these two groups differed with respect to gender, education, health variables, and past experience. Gender (male or female) by adherence (yes or no) is another example of a 2 × 2 chi-square analysis. Education level by adherence is an example of a 3 × 2 chi-square analysis. You can also do 4 × 2 or 3 × 3 analyses, provided you have a minimum of five cases for each cell.

t-Tests

As table 7.1 shows, chi-square analysis is not appropriate for analyzing continuous variables, such as age, number of health problems, or baseline activity level. To compare adherers and dropouts on these continuous variables, use a simple *t*-test, specifically an unpaired *t*-test. Unpaired *t*-tests can compare whether the mean values of *two groups* at one point in time are significant. Paired *t*-tests, on the other hand, compare the mean values on a given variable for a *single group* at two different time points (for instance, when comparing pre- and postassessments for outcome evaluation). If you are comparing the means of more than two groups, or at more than two points in time, you will need to use analysis of variance (ANOVA) rather than a *t*-test. Recall that tables in introductory statistics books will show you whether resulting *t*-test results are statistically significant; the same is true for correlations discussed below.

Correlations

The third comparative statistical procedure to become familiar with is the correlation. Correlations examine the relationship between two variables across clients. For instance, you may want to determine whether age or number of health problems is related to attendance, or whether attendance is related to amount of improvement (on fitness scores, well-being, and so on). The Pearson correlation statistic is the one you will want when comparing continuous variables (e.g., attendance rate and fitness score). The Spearman correlation statistic is intended to compare rank-ordered, categorical variables (e.g., level of education and level of physical activity).

When you tell the computer to compute a correlation, you will obtain an *r*-statistic (or correlation coefficient) as well as a significance level (as described in the previous section). The *r*-value will tell you the strength of the relationship. Correlation coefficients can range from $r = .00$ (indicating no relationship) to $r = 1.00$ (indicating a perfect relationship). What you usually find is a value in between. The rule of thumb is that $r < .30$ indicates a weak association, $r > .30$ but $< .80$ indicates a moderate association, and $r > .80$ indicates a strong association.

The correlation coefficient may have a negative sign (e.g., $r = -.75$) indicating an inverse relationship between the two variables. For instance, age and physical activity tend to be

Table 7.1 Comparison of Adherers and Dropouts

Characteristic	Adherers N = 120	Dropouts N = 50	Statistic	Significance
Gender males females	55 (46%) 65 (54%)	25 (50%) 25 (50%)	Chi-square	NS
Mean age range	29.4 18 to 40	38.6 20 to 69	t-test	$p < .01$
Education college high school less than high school	82 (68%) 25 (21%) 13 (11%)	10 (20%) 19 (38%) 21 (42%)	Chi-square	$p < .01$
Smoker no yes	110 (92%) 10 (8%)	28 (56%) 22 (44%)	Chi-square	$p < .05$
Number of health problems (mean)	1.12	3.42	t-test	$p < .001$
Health limitations no/temporary yes	100 (83%) 20 (17%)	21 (42%) 29 (58%)	Chi-square	$p < .05$
Baseline activity (# days a week) mean range	4.23 3 to 7	1.67 0 to 4	t-test	$p < .01$
Experience no yes, this class yes, similar class	25 (21%) 33 (27%) 62 (52%)	33 (66%) 7 (14%) 10 (20%)	Chi-square	$p < .05$
Reservations mean number range	0.5 0 to 2	1.8 0 to 4	t-test	$p < .05$

inversely related—the older people are, the less likely they are to be highly active. A negative correlation tells you that as the values of one variable to up, the values of the second variable tend to go down. A positive correlation, meanwhile, is when the values of both variables go in the same direction (either both go up or both go down). A good example of a positive association is age and health problems. Older people tend to have more health problems.

Formulas

In addition to the simple statistical procedures described above, your data software program should allow you to enter your own formulas. For evaluation, you are most likely to use formulas to calculate membership growth and attrition across your facility, attendance rates, dropout rates, and client change on outcome measures. You may also need to use formulas to calculate the measure score itself (e.g., BMI or body mass index).

Possible formulas for calculating membership growth, average length of membership, and attrition rate are presented in chapter 3. For instance, the formula for membership growth may be as simple as adding the number of new members who join over a given period (one month, quarterly, or one year) and subtracting the number of terminations over the same period.

You can calculate participation rate based on the number of sessions attended divided by the total number of sessions offered, multiplied by 100 (to obtain a percent). You may decide to do this class by class or across classes of the same type, on a monthly or yearly basis. Computers can easily do these calculations for you, but you must specify the formula you want the computer program to use.

Recall that you must decide on the criteria for absence or dropout. Let's say that for a class that you offer three times a week, you decide to flag participants if they miss six consecutive sessions. Using the spreadsheet example in worksheet 7.3, you would flag clients 3, 5, 9, and 14 for follow-up phone calls by staff. If your definition had been different (e.g., missing nine consecutive sessions), then you would not have flagged client 14, because he or she returned to the class after missing six classes. In this simple example, with only a few clients and a small number of sessions, it is easy to flag absent members visually from the spreadsheet or from the original class attendance sheets. However, as the number of participants and the number of sessions increase, it is easier to let the computer identify absentees for you by entering the formula you choose to define absence or dropout. Once defined, you can use the other statistical tools to determine patterns, such as proportion of dropouts during the first few weeks

of a program, and to profile dropouts (as in table 7.1).

Another formula concerns client change. Recall that for outcome evaluation, you want to collect pre- and postassessments for at least 30 clients on your primary measures. Such measures could include a combination of fitness assessments, performance measures, and self-report measures of functioning or well-being. You could do a paired *t*-test that tells you whether the average change from pre- to postassessment is significant for your sample as a whole.

However, programs tend to be *relatively beneficial*—beneficial for some clients more than for others—depending on the client's baseline level, rate of participation, and so on. Comparing a group's average or means at two points in time (via the *t*-test) will not tell you which clients change or how much each client changes. The following formula enables you to calculate individual client change for each measure:

[(Follow-up – baseline score)
÷ baseline score] × 100
= individual client change

This formula was used by Lord et al. (1996) to examine changes in gait patterns. We have used this formula to examine recovery of injured workers (Williams and Myers 1998a); changes in balance confidence following exercise participation and hip and knee replacement surgery (Myers et al. 1998); changes in mobility, strength, and flexibility in exercising nursing home residents (Lazowski et al. in press); and changes in Vitality Plus Scale (VPS) scale scores following exercise participation (Myers et al. in press).

To give you a more specific illustration, look at the spreadsheet on hypothetical VPS scores in worksheet 7.4. A visual examination of the 15 total scores for T1 and T2 suggests that some clients may have improved and others have not. A *t*-test will give you only the overall mean or average at each time point, because everyone's scores are combined. The formula allows you to further examine the percentage of improvement on an individual client basis.

By using this formula, you can determine the number (and proportion) of clients who deteriorate (negative change), stay the same (0 change), and who improve. You can then look at the range of improvement and the characteristics of clients who improved versus those who did not. For example, which clients lost at least 10 percent of their baseline weight? Which clients lost 20 percent or more? This calculation is useful for identifying the types of clients who show the most improvement from exercise regimens. On the basis of such results, the program may decide to retarget the program or to implement additional activities for clients who tend not to improve.

Williams and Myers (1998a) found that the sample of injured workers improved overall after three weeks in the rehabilitation clinic (paired t-test was significant). Individual change scores showed that 25 percent of this sample did not improve. However, almost 70 percent improved by at least 10 percent (of these, half improved by more than 50 percent, and one client improved by more than 300 percent from clinic entry). In another study, home care clients as a group did not appear to have changed after four months of home exercise (mobility mean scores were comparable at baseline and follow-up, and the t-test was not significant). Keep in mind, this is a declining population. When individual change was examined, 41 percent of the clients were found to decline; however, 59 percent either maintained or improved their mobility scores (Jones et al. 1997). In fact, 36 percent improved by more than 10 percent since starting the exercise regimen.

Analyzing Qualitative Data

As noted at the outset of this chapter, you are most likely to encounter qualitative, or nonnumerical, data in the following situations:

- Responses to open-ended questions on background questionnaires, such as, "How did you hear about the program?"
- Telephone surveys, such as reasons for absence.
- Client-satisfactions surveys, such as, "What did you like most about the program?" or "If you could change one thing about the program, what would it be?"
- Focus groups.

The first three situations are similar, and data analysis consists of simple content analysis. Analysis of focus group data requires several steps and therefore, I discuss it separately.

Content Analysis

Open-ended questions generate either written responses, in the case of a paper-and-pencil questionnaire, or oral responses, in the case of a structured interview. Both written responses and oral responses are likely to be brief, often consisting of single words or short phrases. The purpose of content analysis is to examine and categorize such responses.

Let's take the example of a possible open-ended question on a client-satisfaction survey: "What do you like most about the program?" Let's say that you had 100 completed surveys to work with. To do a content analysis manually, you would need to go through each survey, one at a time, and record the exact (verbatim) response by each person to this question. Next, you would go through this list and look for common types of responses.

For instance, some people may have written "the instructor," others may have written "the group leader," others may have referred to their instructor by name. Because all these responses imply the same thing, you could create a response category labeled "Instructor." A second category that might emerge could be "Social." For instance, people might respond "the other people," or "fellowship," or "the other gals in the class." A third category may be references to the music: "I like the upbeat music," or "the old songs," or "the songs bring back memories," and so on. You need to decide whether you should group all these responses under a single category (e.g., "Music") or under subcategories (e.g., "Music type" and "Music tempo").

You may need to go through the list of verbatim comments several times to develop your coding categories. Once you have created your categories, you can go back through the questionnaires and do a frequency count of the number of times each is mentioned. Often your totals will not add up to the number of survey respondents, because people may provide more than one response to a question. Note that you will have to go through this procedure for each open-ended question on your survey.

When you do a frequency count of written or verbal comments, you are essentially transforming qualitative data into quantitative data. You will probably report such data in rank order, from most to least frequently reported responses. For instance, when asked what they like most about the program, the most common response was the instructor (mentioned by 61 percent), followed by social (50 percent), music (43 percent), and flexible scheduling (24 percent). As another example, the prototype background questionnaire (worksheet 6.4) contains several questions that require content analysis. Question 10, the list of diagnosed health problems, provides the last option "Other health problems? What are they?" Now refer to the codebook (worksheet 7.1) for examples of possible responses, such as Cancer, Epilepsy, Parkinson's, Other (blank). As you code each questionnaire, you can add to this list each time a different health problem is mentioned. You must decide whether to group certain types of responses together (e.g., all forms of cancer) or list them separately (each type of cancer). You might also decide to have a miscellaneous category, because many different but infrequently mentioned problems may emerge. Other examples of coding responses to open-ended questions are provided in the codebook for questions: B11 (type of medications), C15 (what people say they usually do in their leisure time), and D27 (how they heard about this class or program).

With such a large volume of data, let the computer do the work for you. You still must decide on coding categories and variable labels. However, the computer's analytical tools can do the frequency counts and rankings. Furthermore, you may want to make comparisons. For instance, you might want to look at whether people who say they heard about the program through word of mouth (question D27) are more likely to know someone in the program (question D28). A chi-square analysis would be appropriate here. You might want to examine whether people who heard about the program on the radio (question D27) are older (question A2). You would compute the mean age of those who heard about the program on the radio versus other ways, and use a *t*-test to determine whether the two groups differ significantly in age.

Focus Group Data

As described in chapter 6, there are several pieces of data in focus groups that you need to analyze: field notes, debriefing notes, the taped discussion session, and possibly information from background questionnaires.

A background questionnaire provides a description of your sample, such as gender, age, level of experience (length of time in the program), and so on. Some information, such as number of males and females in the group, is apparent, and you are likely to record it in the seating plan. You may solicit experience with the program or issue under discussion through the discussion itself, perhaps in the icebreaker question. Whether or not you administer a background questionnaire, you will still need to provide a general description of your recruitment process and the composition of each focus group.

Recall that *field notes* are recorded observations of the session and the participants. For instance, the recorder might make notes on who spoke the most (or least); nonverbal gestures, such as head nodding during certain parts of the discussion; unique characteristics, such as only one person had prior experience; and so on.

Debriefing takes place immediately following each session. Together, the facilitator and recorder discuss their impressions. You can either take notes or tape-record the debriefing conversation. This is essentially your first step at data analysis—your initial impressions of the major themes or issues that emerged from the discussion. What are the things that stood out most? What were the major areas of agreement and disagreement? What things did participants feel most strongly about?

In-depth analysis takes place using the tape recording of the session. Analysis of focus group data is *different* from doing a content analysis on short responses to open-ended survey questions. With focus group data, don't isolate short phrases or do frequency counts. Keep people's comments in context. By reducing the discussion to single words or phrases, you will lose the richness and meaning of what participants are saying. Keep in mind that people's opinions may change during the course of the discussion and in light of comments made by other participants.

Focus group data requires *thematic analysis*. Basically, you are searching for the primary

Table 7.2 Transcription From Focus Group With Older Men's Fitness Program

Facilitator: What keeps you coming back to your program?

Bill: The fellowship. The fact that when we're here for a short time we're walking with somebody and we're getting into conversation, and you learn something about what the person is doing, or a lot of us talking politics or everything under the sun and you can exchange viewpoints. It keeps your mind very active, and I think that the camaraderie and the friendship is the principal reason we're sticking together here. And I really know this sounds controversial but the physical part of it is secondary. Although we enjoy it; we enjoy being fitter than we would be if we weren't in (the class). I don't know if anyone wants to disagree with me or not.

Andrew: I disagree with Bill a little bit 'cause it's the physical thing (that) is the foundation on which I'm here, and from what I'm hearing most of us are here because of our concern about our physical condition. But there is no question about it, the camaraderie and the discussion we have and the joke telling and all the rest of it holds us together as well. And it must do very well because we've gone through some adversity as far as the hour we start, the place we work; we've had all kinds of disagreeable things that probably have caused some people to leave our group. But I think that the majority of us stick despite these problems.

Phil: I think the facilities themselves are a great asset here . . . and the parking is close and (the program) is organized so you just fall into (the routine). It's very good . . . . I see people in the mall but that's secondary to what we have.

Facilitator: Why do you say that?

Phil: Because we have a tremendous track . . . and that helps for the aging process, people's knees and the rest, you know.

themes, issues, or ideas that emerge from the discussion. Following the script, examine each question or topic sequentially. Then look at the discussion as a whole to examine whether certain themes or viewpoints came up throughout or whether people's opinions changed as the discussion evolved.

You can conduct your thematic analysis simply by listening to the audiotape several times, but it is easier to work with a typed transcription. A transcript is a verbatim (word by word) write-up of everything participants said in the discussion session. If the recorder made notes during the session on each speaker (and their first few words), it is easy to insert this information into the transcription. Table 7.2 shows you a partial transcription from an actual focus group conducted with 12 men (mean age = 70) participating in an older men's fitness program with 100 members—the Men's Retirement Association. The aim of this focus group was to explore why this model was successful in maintaining

such a large membership base for nearly two decades. Note that each comment is attributed to a particular speaker (but real names are not used to protect confidentiality).

When you work with a transcription, you can make notes in the margins, photocopy and cut and paste different sections to rearrange the text, or use highlighted pens to identify themes (each highlighted with a different color), subthemes, and possible quotations you may want to use in your write-up. You can enter transcribed text into the computer if you want to use a qualitative software package such as NUD*IST to assist with data analysis. A program like NUD*IST allows you to move text around, search, index, and display text (Richards and Richards 1991).

Whether you are working with a transcript or the original audiotape, the facilitator and the assistant (or another person) should conduct the thematic analysis separately. If the two parties independently find the same results, you have more confidence in the findings. If a sample of partici-

Table 7.3 Themes Emerging From Focus Groups With Older Men's Fitness Program

Emerging themes	Example quotes
Vulnerability	"I felt that this should be a good way of keeping fit and in reasonable condition as you are aging. Because I could feel it at this age that I was, uh, deteriorating rather rapidly. That is, I would go out and dig a little bit and I'd have a sore back." "I go to church and I see these people. You know, they can hardly walk. I think a lot of it is because they haven't done anything. You know, they just sit and they can't move after a while."
Purpose	"The regimentation of getting you up in the morning, three mornings a week, keeping you at it, is good. Otherwise you tend to, in the wintertime, if you don't do something like this, you tend to roll over and say the hell with it." "I think it puts regularity in your life. You know, there's three mornings in a week where you have to get up and have to go and that sets a lifestyle for the week, and I think that the regularity of it is important because when you retire if you don't have specific things to do at a specific time, you have a tendency to become a couch potato."
Social interaction	"The fact that when we're here for a short time we're walking with somebody and we're getting into conversation, and you learn something about what the person is doing, or a lot of us talking politics or everything under the sun and you can exchange viewpoints. It keeps your mind very active." "And it's also very . . . I don't know how to explain this . . . but it's very important that we are fairly ancient and yet . . . have young women, or young people (instructing), and it's something that kind of keeps us in touch with other than our own age group, but on a pleasant level, and it's something very positive about having young women as our exercise leaders."

pants themselves also agree with the findings, confidence is further increased. As described in chapter 6, obtain consent to later contact a few people from each group to verify your primary findings.

Start your search for themes question by question or issue by issue (following your script). Then look at the discussion as a whole to see how things tie together and whether people's opinions changed as the discussion evolved. Once you have thoroughly analyzed each focus group session, compare findings across groups. Was group composition similar? Did the same themes emerge? Was the pattern of agreement or disagreement similar? Recall that you should conduct at least two focus groups for a given evaluation project. Once the same themes begin to emerge repeatedly, or become repetitive (termed *saturation*),

it is unlikely that conducting further groups on the same topic will reveal any new information.

Table 7.3 provides an example of three major themes that emerged from the Men's Retirement Association's fitness program focus group (Tudor-Locke and Myers 1998). We found it particularly interesting that the program hires primarily young female instructors and chooses to keep their group restricted to retired males. Sure enough, there were two subthemes under the third category, social interaction—camaraderie with the other men in the program and interaction with the young instructors. The more recent members repeatedly commented on the strength of the bonds they observed in the group and how everyone encouraged each other (especially on cold mornings). This feature of the group was something they valued and wanted to be part of. Table 7.3 provides illustrative quotations for each theme, similar to what you might include in an evaluation report.

Reporting and Presenting Findings

When data analysis is completed, your remaining tasks are to document the findings, develop recommendations, and decide how to report or present this information. Each evaluation project or activity has a purpose, as well as an intended audience or intended users. Often, the purpose is directly tied to the intended users of the evaluation information.

Let's refer to the scenarios again. The reason for doing evaluation, as well as the evaluation approach, differed for each scenario. Each case has its own intended users or audience for the evaluation findings. For instance, the rehabilitation clinic in scenario 5 (p. 8) was asked to provide indicators of recovery by the workers' compensation board, who funds and accredits this private clinic. The recreation director in scenario 6 (p. 8) wanted to convince the nursing home administrator and medical director that more challenging exercise programming is both feasible and beneficial for the residents. The health educators in scenarios 2 (p. 7) and 4 (p. 7), working with the textile plant and the mall-walking program, respectively, would both have to report to their public health unit administrators. The personal trainer in scenario 9 (p. 9) planned to use his evaluation findings to obtain more physician referrals to increase his client base. In several other scenarios—the director of occupational health and safety (scenario 1, p. 6), the YMCA manager (scenario 3, p. 7), and the director of the senior's center (scenario 8, p. 9)—the directors

Worksheet 7.5
Template for Evaluation Reports

I. Executive Summary
- Two- to three-page overview of the project
- Written in nontechnical language

II. Description of the Program
- Program components, activities, and materials
- Objectives (logic model if possible)
- Target audience or clientele
- Staffing and operation

III. Purpose of the Project
- Rationale and evaluation approach(es)

IV. Data-Collection Procedures
- Outline each strategy (attach tools used)
- Outline recruitment or sampling procedures

V. Findings
- Describe the response rate and sample characteristics
- Present descriptive, followed by comparative, quantitative findings
- Present emerging themes with illustrative quotes for focus group data
- Display results simply and visually (tables and graphs)

VI. Conclusions and Recommendations
- Discuss each important finding with respect to project rationale, strengths, and limitations
- Provide support or evidence for each recommendation

themselves are the primary intended users of the evaluation findings.

Even if you are doing evaluation to inform your own decision making, you should still document your findings for future reference in case you later need to justify your decisions. Most likely, you will want to share your findings with your colleagues in your facility or agency to get their feedback. For instance, the YMCA manager may not make the decision of whether to offer a new Tai Chi program on his own. He probably would share the needs assessment findings and his recommendations with his colleagues before making any final decisions. If the evaluation project has been a team effort, then all the team members should review and comment on the findings.

Thus, in some instances, you may be *asked* to share your evaluation findings and recommendations (for instance with upper level management). In other cases, you will be *expected* to share your findings (e.g., for accreditation purposes). Many times, you simply *want* to share your findings to justify your program, argue for increased resources, or to brainstorm with your colleagues and obtain their input.

Whether you present your evaluation findings orally, in a written report, or both, start with an outline for your report or presentation. Worksheet 7.5 contains a template describing the six primary sections that you should include in written evaluation reports.

The *executive summary*, although only a few pages, is the most important section of any report. This section provides a brief overview of the evaluation project's purpose, methods, primary findings, and recommendations. Some people may read only the executive summary, or may make a judgement based on this summary of whether they want to read more of the report. Write this section carefully, and last—after producing the other sections of the report.

The remaining five sections should guide both written and oral presentations of evaluation findings. Depending on your audience, each section may require more or less detail. When preparing for oral presentations, allow enough time—about 20 percent to 25 percent total presentation time—for questions and comments.

Tailoring the Presentation

You may be asked or want to give a copy of the report or make a presentation to several different groups (for example, fitness instructors, man-agers, boards of directors, the membership, or referring physicians). Be sure to tailor your report and presentation to each audience. Consider how much the audience already knows about

- the program in question;
- evaluation in general, and the specific approach to evaluation used in this project;
- the purposes of this evaluation project; and
- the data-collection and analysis strategies used in the evaluation.

For instance, if your audience is familiar with the program, you don't need to describe it in great detail. You may wish, however, to show them the logic model that illustrates the links among program components, activities, and objectives. Although your audience may be familiar with the program, they may not have experience with evaluation. In this case, you may need to explain the specific approach you are using (needs assessment, process, or outcome).

Ideally, key stakeholders or primary intended users have been involved in the evaluation project since the original planning or proposal stage. For this audience, they already know the rationale or purpose of the project. Similarly, they will have had direct input concerning the proposed approach, data-collection strategies, and sampling procedures. Ideally, you will have kept them informed of the project's progress and any departures (changes in data-collection procedures) from the proposal. When presenting the findings, you may need to give a brief overview of the methods simply to refresh their memories, but there should be no surprises, especially if you have shown them the evaluation plan and given them periodic progress reports, including preliminary findings.

Explain data-collection and sampling procedures clearly and simply. Once again, consider your audience's familiarity with the methods used (e.g., focus groups, telephone surveys, specific fitness assessments, or psychological inventories). Attach copies of your tools (e.g., focus group protocol and script, background questionnaire, telephone survey protocol, outcome measures) for written reports. Use simple overheads (e.g., the focus group script) when verbally describing the procedure. Recall that people are more likely to challenge your findings if they are unfamiliar with the methods used to collect the data. For instance, at the end of a presentation on focus group themes, someone may ask, "But, where are the numbers?"

Preempt such challenges by explaining and justifying data-collection methods *before* presenting your results. Tailor length and detail of method explanation based on audience familiarity.

Executing the Presentation

Presenting the findings of an evaluation project is usually the most difficult part of evaluation reporting. First, it is important to always put your sampling in context. For instance, let's say that you plan to report the findings of 100 client-satisfaction surveys. How many participants were present the days you conducted the survey? What proportion completed the survey? What percentage of the total membership does this represent?

You can put details of the analyses into an appendix of a report (or in a separate technical report), or hand them out as a supplement following a presentation. Only a few people are likely to be interested in statistical values. However, such results should be available for those who are interested (or those who may wish to scrutinize your analyses). In the body of a report or in an oral presentation, you want to present the main findings in a simple and logical order. For quantitative data, present descriptive results before comparative results. Present themes emerging from focus groups with illustrative quotes (see table 7.3).

Present results in summary form, either in tables or graphs. Tables are useful for presenting results such as client-satisfaction ratings (as illustrated by table 3.2) or group comparisons on a number of variables (as illustrated by table 7.1). Remember, in Western cultures, people read from left to right, so set up the information accordingly.

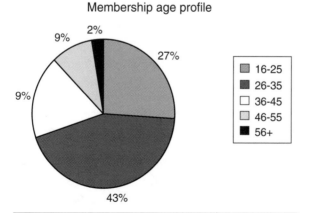

Membership age profile

Figure 7.2 Microsoft Excel pie chart.

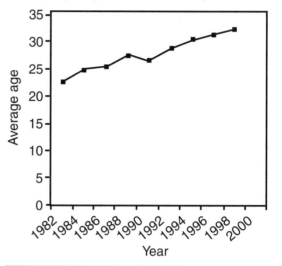

Average age of membership 1982-2000

Figure 7.3 A trend graph.

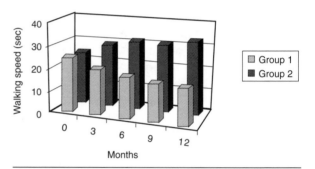

Figure 7.4 A bar graph.

Many people process information visually, but be wary of information overload! Don't put too much information in a single table or graph. Nothing is worse than looking at an overhead that is cluttered and so small that no one in the audience can possibly read the numbers.

Some information lends itself to graphical display for presentation, for reports, overheads, or slides, and you can create them in the same software you used to analyze the data. For example, figure 7.2, which profiles membership ages, was created using Microsoft Excel.

Pie charts are an excellent way of illustrating distributions in terms of age, education level, financial status, or other characteristics of either potential or current clientele. If you want to show results over time, such as client-satisfaction ratings year by year, or changing profiles of membership, a trend graph is a good choice. Figure 7.3 illustrates that this club's membership has steadily increased in age since the 1980s.

A bar graph is a useful way of illustrating group differences on a single measure over time or on multiple measures at one point in time. The example in figure 7.4 shows a three-dimensional picture of walking speed for two groups over a 12-month period. The graph indicates that, although the two groups were comparable at baseline, scores for Group 1 have steadily increased, and scores for Group 2 have steadily decreased.

Your audience will need to know more about the measures to interpret these findings; walk them through the results. In this example, we used the self-paced walk test (Himann et al. 1988). Participants were asked to walk four lengths of a 20-meter course at three speeds—slow, normal, and fast. Figure 7.4 presents the results of the fast-paced walking speed. According to the developers' instructions, higher scores indicate poor mobility (such individuals take longer to complete the course or have slower walking speeds). Walking speeds of 20 seconds or longer (20 seconds is approximately equal to one meter per second) indicate impaired mobility. Such individuals may be in jeopardy of crossing a street safely (Himann et al. 1988). Figure 7.4 shows that Group 2 is deteriorating over time. This group might be frail or have a chronic health condition that impairs their mobility. Group 1, however, is steadily improving, as a result of the exercise intervention.

The final section of an evaluation report or presentation is usually the most interesting. Here is where you present the bottom line. What can you conclude from your evaluation findings? How confident are you in drawing these conclusions? What are the implications for the program? Recommendations for the program in question should follow from the evaluation findings. For instance, based on the findings, you may conclude that your program is reaching its intended target audience and recommend that you continue to use current recruitment procedures. Conversely, your findings may suggest that potential consumers are not aware of the program, and you may need to develop new advertising strategies. If you obtained in-depth feedback from potential consumers (for instance through focus

groups), you may have concrete suggestions for particular advertising strategies.

Findings from a process evaluation may indicate that the proportion of older adults in your membership has increased. Such findings may lead you to consider offering alternate programming (such as low- versus high-impact aerobics classes) for this segment. Or, results from an outcome evaluation may indicate that certain clients benefit more from structured classes than from unstructured workouts. You may recommend encouraging clients to join classes, during the initial consultation and appraisal.

Evaluation is the basis for *informed* decision making. It is much easier to convince other stakeholders to start a new program, expand or modify an existing program, or discontinue a service, if you have evidence to back up your recommendations.

Summary

I hope this book has convinced you that all types of exercise programs can benefit from doing program evaluation. If you are considering offering a new program, service, or exercise equipment, conducting a needs assessment will help you determine what clients want out of a new program. Market testing with potential consumers will help you develop effective advertising strategies, program materials, and scheduling that meets the expectations of your target group. Implementation evaluation helps keep you on track.

Once the program is operational, process evaluation becomes the priority. You likely already conduct periodic client-satisfaction surveys. Now you can complement such surveys with more in-depth feedback through focus groups. You likely know how many clients are in your program. Now you can obtain a more detailed profile of your clientele; compare frequent and infrequent users, adherers and dropouts; and track patterns over time. Such information will help you to better serve your clientele.

Most of you routinely conduct individual client-fitness appraisals. Outcome evaluation simply entails comparing baseline (or preassessment) and follow-up (or postassessment) scores after some period of participation. Furthermore, you want to make these comparisons across your clientele to determine how many improve, how much they improve, and which types of clients improve the most. You can still promote your programs through success stories, but now your success stories, put in context, will be more believable.

Evaluation will give your exercise program, service, or facility the competitive edge in the marketplace—a marketplace that is increasing steadily and will continue to increase over the upcoming decades. Unless you have a magic crystal ball, evaluation will allow you track patterns, obtain the input of current and potential consumers, and make informed projections.

Don't try to do everything at once. Start by defining your priority areas—your most important and timely needs for evaluation. Choose one evaluation project and follow the steps outlined in this book. Use the tools provided by the worksheets to get started. Modify these tools to meet your informational needs. Choose from the outcome tools described in chapter 5. Follow the steps in chapters 6 and 7 for conducting focus groups and analyzing your findings. Your confidence will increase with each effort. You do *not* have to be a researcher or a statistician. Anyone can do evaluation and everyone should. Using this resource as you undertake each evaluation project, you will see that the rewards of program evaluation are well worth the effort.

References

American College of Sports Medicine (ACSM). 1978. Position statement on the recommended quantity and quality of exercise for developing and maintaining fitness in healthy adults. *Medicine and Science in Sports and Exercise* 10:7-10.

———. 1990. The recommended quantity and quality of exercise for developing and maintaining cardiorespiratory and muscular fitness in healthy adults: Position stand. *Medicine and Science in Sports and Exercise* 22:265-274.

———. 1995. *ACSM's guidelines for exercise testing and prescription*. 5th ed. Boston: Williams and Wilkins.

———. 1997a. *ACSM's health/fitness facility standards and guidelines*. 2nd ed. Champaign, IL: Human Kinetics.

———. 1997b. *ACSM's exercise management for persons with chronic diseases and disabilities*. Champaign, IL: Human Kinetics.

———. 1998a. The recommended quantity and quality of exercise for developing and maintaining cardiorespiratory and muscular fitness, and flexibility in healthy adults: Position stand. *Medicine and Science in Sports and Exercise* 30:975-991.

———. 1998b. Exercise and physical activity for older adults. *Medicine and Science in Sports and Exercise* 30:992-1008.

American College of Sports Medicine (ACSM) and American Diabetes Association (ADA). 1997. Joint position statement: Diabetes mellitus and exercise. *Medicine and Science in Sports and Exercise* 29:1-6.

Armitage, P., and B. Berry. 1987. *Statistical methods in medical research*. 2nd ed. Oxford: Blackwell Scientific.

Bandura, A. 1977. Self-efficacy: Toward a unifying theory of behavioral change. *Psychological Review* 84:191-215.

———. 1997. *Self-efficacy: The exercise of control*. New York: W.H. Freeman.

Berg, K., S. Wood-Dauphinee, J.I. Williams, and D. Gayton. 1989. Measuring balance in the elderly: Preliminary development of an instrument. *Physiotherapy Canada* 41:304-311.

Bouchard, C., A. Tremblay, C. LeBlanc, G. Lortie, R. Savard, and G. Theriault. 1983. A method to assess energy expenditure in children and adults. *American Journal of Clinical Nutrition* 37:461-467.

Brassington, G.S., and R.A. Hicks. 1995. Aerobic exercise and self-reported sleep quality in elderly individuals. *Journal of Aging and Physical Activity* 3:120-134.

Brooks, C. 1994. *How consumers view health and sports clubs*. Ann Arbor, MI: International Health, Racquet, and Sports Club Association.

Browne, D.W. 1984. Reduced disability and health care costs in an industrial fitness program. *Journal of Occupational Medicine* 26:809-816.

Buysse, D.J., C.F. Reynolds, T.H. Monk, S.R. Berman, and D.J. Kupfer. 1989. The Pittsburgh Sleep Quality Index: A new instrument for psychiatric practice and research. *Psychiatry Research* 28:193-213.

Canadian Fitness and Lifestyles Research Institute (CFLRI). 1996a. *How active are Canadians?* Bulletin no. 1. Ottawa, ON: Canadian Fitness and Lifestyles Research Institute.

———. 1996b. *The economics of participation*. Bulletin no. 10. Ottawa, ON: Canadian Fitness and Lifestyles Research Institute.

———. 1996c. *Location for physical activity*. Bulletin no. 12. Ottawa, ON: Canadian Fitness and Lifestyles Research Institute.

———. 1996d. *Barriers to physical activity*. Bulletin no. 4. Ottawa, ON: Canadian Fitness and Lifestyles Research Institute.

Canadian Physiotherapy Association (CPA). 1994. *Physical rehabilitation outcome measures*. Ottawa, ON: Supply and Services Canada and the Canadian Physiotherapy Association.

Canadian Society for Exercise Physiology (CSEP). 1996. *The Canadian physical activity, fitness and lifestyle appraisal: CSEP's guide to healthy active living*. Ottawa, ON: Canadian Society for Exercise Physiology.

Carron, A.V., W.N. Widmeyer, and L.R. Brawley. 1988. Group cohesion and individual adherence to physical activity. *Journal of Sport and Exercise Psychology* 10:127-138.

Caspersen, C.J., K.E. Powell, and G.M. Christensen. 1985. Physical activity, exercise and physical fitness: Definitions and distinctions for health-related research. *Public Health Reports* 100:126-130.

Clark, D.O. 1996. Age, socioeconomic status, and exercise self-efficacy. *The Gerontologist* 36:157-164.

Cotton, R.T., C.J. Ekeroth, and H. Yancy, eds. 1998. *Exercise for older adults: ACE's guide for fitness professionals*. Champaign, IL: Human Kinetics.

Courneya, K.S., and E. McAuley. 1995. Reliability and discriminant validity of subjective norm, social support, and cohesion in an exercise setting. *Journal of Sport and Exercise Psychology* 17:325-337.

Desrosiers, J., A. Rochette, H. Payette, L. Gregoire, V. Boutier, and D.A. Lazowski. 1998. Upper extremity isometric strength measurement using the belt-resisted method. *Canadian Journal of Rehabilitation* 11:143-149.

Dillman, D. 1978. *Mail and telephone surveys: The total design method*. Toronto: John Wiley and Sons.

Dishman, R.K., ed. 1994. *Advances in exercise adherence*. Champaign, IL: Human Kinetics.

Dishman, R.K., and S.F. Sallis. 1994. Determinants and interventions for physical activity and exercise. In *Physical activity, fitness, and health: International proceedings and consensus statement*, edited by C. Bouchard, R. Shepard, and T. Stephens. Champaign, IL: Human Kinetics.

Duncan, P.W., D.K. Weiner, J. Chandler, and S. Studenski. 1990. Functional reach: A new clinical measure of balance. *Journal of Gerontology: Medical Sciences* 45:M192-M197.

Ecclestone, N.A., A.M. Myers, and D.H. Patterson. 1998. Tracking older participants of twelve physical activity classes over a three-year period. *Journal of Aging and Physical Activity* 6:70-82.

Ewart, C.K., K.J. Stewart, R.E. Gillilan, and M.H. Kelemen. 1986. Self-efficacy mediates strength gains during circuit weight training in men with coronary artery disease. *Medicine and Science in Sports and Exercise* 18:531-540.

Favaro, P. 1995. Consumer satisfaction with mental health services: Methodological, measurement and practical issues. In *Evaluation methods sourcebook II*, edited by A. J. Love. Ottawa, ON: Evaluation Society Press.

Ferrini, A.F., and R.L. Ferrini. 1993. *Health in the later years*. 2nd ed. Madison, WI: Wm. C. Brown.

Foot, D.K. 1996. *Boom, bust, and echo*. Toronto: Macfarlane, Walter and Ross.

Frisancho, A.R. 1990. *Anthropometric standards for the assessment of growth and nutritional status*. Ann Arbor, MI: University of Michigan Press.

Fry, E. 1977. Fry's readability graph: Clarifications, validity, and extension to level 17. *Journal of Reading* 20: 242-252.

Gauvin, L., and W.J. Rejeski. 1993. The Exercise-Induced Feeling Inventory: Development and initial validation. *Journal of Sport and Exercise Psychology* 15:403-423.

Granger, C.V., and B.B. Hamilton. 1993. Performance profiles of the Functional Independence Measure. *Archives of Physical Medicine and Rehabilitation* 72:84-89.

Grantham, W.C., R.W. Patton, T.D. York, and M.L. Winick. 1998. *Health fitness management*. Champaign, IL: Human Kinetics.

Gray, E., and A.M. Myers. 1997. Evaluation of the HeartMobile health promotion program. *Canadian Journal of Program Evaluation* 12:19-29.

Guralnik, J.M., L.G. Branch, S.R. Cummings, and J.D. Curb. 1989. Physical performance measures in aging research. *Journal of Gerontology: Medical Sciences* 44:M141-M146.

Harada, M. 1994. Early and later life sport participation patterns among the active elderly in Japan. *Journal of Aging and Physical Activity* 2:105-114.

Hatziandreu, E.I. 1988. A cost-effectiveness analysis of exercise as health promotion activity. *American Journal of Public Health* 78:1417-1421.

Helmes, E., A. Hodsman, D.A. Lazowski, A. Bhardwaj, R. Crilly, P. Nichol, D. Drost, L. Vanderburgh, and L. Pederson. 1995. A questionnaire to evaluate disability in osteoporotic patients with vertebral compression fractures. *Journal of Gerontology: Medical Sciences* 50A:M91-M98.

Hillsdon, M., and M. Thorogood. 1996. A systematic review of physical activity promotion strategies. *British Journal of Sport Medicine* 30:84-89.

Himann, J.E., D.A. Cunningham, P.A. Rechnitzer, and D. Paterson. 1988. Age-related changes in speed of walking. *Medicine and Science in Sports and Exercise* 20:161-166.

Hooke, A.P., and M.B. Zoller. 1992. *Active older adults in the YMCA: A resource manual*. Champaign, IL: Human Kinetics.

Hudson, J., J. Mayne, and R. Thomlison, eds. 1992. *Action-oriented evaluation in organizations: Canadian practices*. Toronto: Wall & Emerson.

Jones, G.R., N.A. Ecclestone, D.H. Patterson, A.M. Myers, D.A. Lazowski, and C. Tudor-Locke. 1997. Leadership training for exercise programs for frail older adults in long-term care facilities or in homebound settings (abstract). *Journal of Aging and Physical Activity* 5:394.

Jones, R.C., J. Bly, and J. Richardson. 1990. A study of a worksite health promotion program and absenteeism. *Journal of Occupational Medicine* 32: 95-99.

Kaplan, R.M., C.J. Atkins, and S. Reinsch. 1984. Specific exercise expectations mediate exercise compliance in patients with COPD. *Health Psychology* 3: 223-242.

King, A.C., W.L. Haskell, B. Taylor, H.C. Kraemer, and R.F. DeBusk. 1991. Group- vs. home-based exercise training in healthy older men and women: A community-based clinical trial. *Journal of the American Medical Association* 266:1535-1542.

King, A.C., R. F. Oman, G.S. Brassington, D.L. Bliwise, and W.L. Haskell. 1997. Moderate-intensity exercise and self-rated quality of sleep in older adults: A randomized controlled trial. *Journal of the American Medical Association* 277:32-37.

Kotler, P. 1976. *Marketing management*. 3rd ed. Englewood Cliffs, NJ: Prentice Hall.

Kotler, P., and A.R. Anderson. 1987. *Strategic marketing for nonprofit organizations*. Englewood Cliffs, NJ: Prentice Hall.

Kriska, A.M., and P.H. Bennett. 1992. An epidemiological perspective of the relationship between physical activity and NIDDM: From activity assessment to intervention. *Diabetes Metabolism Review* 8:355-372.

Kriska, A.M., and C.J. Caspersen, eds. 1997. A collection of physical activity questionnaires for health-related research. *Medicine and Science in Sports and Exercise* 24 (Suppl.): S1-S205.

Krueger, R.A. 1994. *Focus groups: A practical guide for applied research*. 2nd ed. Thousand Oaks, CA: Sage.

Krug, L.M., D. Haire-Joshu, and S.A. Heady. 1991. Exercise habits and exercise relapse in persons with non-insulin-dependent diabetes mellitus. *The Diabetes Educator* 17:185-188.

Kvale, S. 1996. *Interviews: An introduction to qualitative research interviewing*. Thousand Oaks, CA: Sage.

Lazowski, D.A., N.A. Ecclestone, A.M. Myers, D.H. Paterson, C. Tudor-Locke, C. Fitzgerald, G. Jones, N. Shima, and D.A. Cunningham. In press. A randomized outcome evaluation of group exercise programs in long-term care institutions. *Journal of Gerontology: Medical Sciences*.

Lazowski, D.A., N.A. Ecclestone, D.H. Paterson, C. Fitzgerald, G. Jones, and C.E. Tudor-Locke. 1997. Using a group exercise program to improve the flexibility of frail older adults living in long-term care institutions. *Journal of Aging and Physical Activity* 5:376.

Lord, S.R., D.G. Lloyd, M. Nirui, J. Raymond, P. Williams, and R.A. Stewart. 1996. The effect of exercise on gait patterns in older women: A randomized trial. *Journal of Gerontology* 51A:M64-M70.

Lorig, K., R.L. Chastain, E. Ung, S. Shoor, and H. Holman. 1989. Development and evaluation of a scale to measure perceived self-efficacy in people with arthritis. *Arthritis and Rheumatism* 32:37-44.

Marcus, B.H., S.W. Banspach, R.C. Lefebvre, J.S. Rossi, R.A. Carleton, and D.B. Abrams. 1992. Using the stages of change model to increase the adoption of physical activity among community participants. *American Journal of Health Promotion* 6:424-429.

McAuley, E., and K.S. Courneya. 1994. The Subjective Exercise Experiences Scale (SEES): Development and validation. *Journal of Sport and Exercise Psychology* 16:163-177.

McAuley, E., and L. Jacobson. 1991. Self-efficacy and exercise participation in sedentary adult females. *American Journal of Health Promotion* 5:185-191.

McAuley, E., C. Lox, and T.E. Duncan. 1993. Long-term maintenance of exercise, self-efficacy, and physiological change in older adults. *Journal of Gerontology: Psychological Sciences* 48:P218-224.

McAuley, E., and D. Rudolph. 1995. Physical activity, aging, and psychological well-being. *Journal of Aging and Physical Activity* 3:67-96.

McDowell, I., and C. Newell. 1996. *Measuring health: A guide to rating scales and questionnaires*. 2nd ed. Toronto: Oxford University Press.

McHorney, C.A. 1996. Measuring and monitoring general health status in elderly persons: Practical and methodological issues in using the SF-36 Health Survey. *The Gerontologist* 36:571-583.

McHorney, C.A., J.E. Ware, and A.E. Raczek. 1993. The MOS 36-item short form health survey (SF-36): II Psychometric and clinical tests of validity in measuring physical and mental health constructs. *Medical Care* 31:247-263.

McLaughlin, G.H. 1969. SMOG grading: A new readability formula. *Journal of Reading* 12:639-646.

Meenan, R.F. 1982. The AIMS approach to health status measurement: Conceptual background and measurement properties. *Journal of Rheumatology* 9:785-788.

Mertens, D.E. 1998. *Research methods in education and psychology: Integrating diversity with quantitative and qualitative approaches*. Thousand Oaks, CA: Sage.

Miller, P.A., ed. 1995. *Fitness programming and physical disability*. Champaign, IL: Human Kinetics.

Minor, M.A., and J.D. Brown. 1993. Exercise maintenance of persons with arthritis after participation in a class experience. *Health Education Quarterly* 20:83-95.

Morgan, D.L. 1993. *Successful focus groups: Advancing the state of the art*. Thousand Oaks, CA: Sage.

Morgan, D.L., and R.A. Krueger. 1998. *The focus group kit*. Thousand Oaks, CA: Sage.

Mullin, B.J., S. Hardy, and W.A. Sutton. 1993. *Sport marketing*. Champaign, IL: Human Kinetics.

Myers, A. M. 1987. Advising your elderly patients concerning safe exercising. *Canadian Family Physician* 33:195-205.

———. 1988. Needs assessment: Broadening the perspective on utility and timing. *Canadian Journal of Program Evaluation* 3:103-113.

———. 1992. Evaluation as an organization process. In *Action-oriented evaluation in organizations: Canadian practices*, edited by J. Hudson, J. Mayne, and R. Thomlison. Toronto: Wall & Emerson.

———. 1996. Coming to grips with changing Canadian health care organizations: Challenges for evaluation. *Canadian Journal of Program Evaluation* 11:127-147.

Myers, A.M., P.C. Fletcher, A.H. Myers, and W. Sherk. 1998. Discriminative and evaluative properties of the Activities-specific Balance Confidence (ABC) Scale. *Journal of Gerontology: Medical Sciences* 53A:M287-M294.

Myers, A.M., and N. Hamilton. 1985. Evaluation of the Canadian Red Cross Society's Fun and Fitness program for seniors. *Canadian Journal on Aging* 4:201-212.

Myers, A.M., P. Holliday, K. Harvey, and K. Hutchinson. 1993. Functional performance measures: Are they superior to self-assessments? *Journal of Gerontology: Medical Sciences* 48:M196-M206.

Myers, A.M., O.W. Malott, E. Gray, C. Tudor-Locke, N.A. Ecclestone, S. O'Brien Cousins, and R. Petrella. In press. Measuring accumulated health-related benefits of exercise participation for older adults: The Vitality Plus Scale. *Journal of Gerontology: Medical Sciences*.

Myers, A.M., L. Powell, B. Maki, P. Holliday, L. Brawley, and W. Sherk. 1996. Psychology of balance confidence: Relationship to actual and perceived abilities. *Journal of Gerontology: Medical Sciences* 51A:M37-43.

Myers, A.M., C. Weigel, and P.J. Holliday. 1989. Sex- and age-linked determinants of physical activity in adulthood. *Canadian Journal of Public Health* 80:256-260.

Newcomer, K.E. 1997. Using performance measurement to improve programs. *New Directions for Program Evaluation* 75:5-13.

O'Brien Cousins, S. 1997. An older adult exercise inventory: Reliability and validity in adults over 70. *Journal of Sport Behaviour* 19:288-306.

———. 1998. *Exercise, aging and health: Overcoming barriers to an active old age*. Philadelphia: Brunner/Mazel.

O'Brien Cousins, S., and A. Burgess. 1992. Perspectives on older adults in physical activity and sports. *Educational Gerontology* 18:461-481.

O'Brien Cousins, S., and T. Horne. 1998. *Active living among older adults: Health benefits and outcomes*. Philadelphia: Brunner/Mazel.

O'Brien Cousins, S., and P.A. Vertinsky. 1991. Unfit survivors: Exercise as a resource for aging women. *The Gerontologist* 31:347-357.

Oldridge, N.B. 1979. Compliance of post myocardial infarction patients to exercise programs. *Medicine and Science in Sports and Exercise* 11:373-375.

———. 1982. Compliance and exercise in primary and secondary prevention of coronary heart disease: A review. *Preventive Medicine* 11:56-70.

Osness, W.H., M. Adrian, B. Clark, W. Hoeger, D. Raab, and R. Wiswell. 1990. *Functional fitness assessment for adults over 60 years (A field based assessment)*. Reston, VA: American Alliance for Health, Physical Education, Recreation and Dance.

Padgett, D.K. 1991. Correlates of self-efficacy beliefs among patients with non-insulin dependent diabetes mellitus in Zagreb, Yugoslavia. *Patient Education and Counselling* 18:139-147.

Pate, R.R., M. Pratt, S. Blair, W. Haskell, C. Macera, C. Bouchard, D. Buchner, W. Ettinger, G. Heath, A. King, A. Kriska, A. Leon, B. Marcus, J. Movis, R. Paffenbarger, K. Patrick, M. Pollack, J. Rippe, J. Sallis, and J. Wilmore. 1995. Physical activity and public health: A recommendation from the Centers for Disease Control and Prevention and the American College of Sports Medicine. *Journal of the American Medical Association* 273:402-407.

Patton, M.Q. 1997. *Utilization-focused evaluation: The new century text*. 3rd ed. Thousand Oaks, CA: Sage.

Podsiadlo, D., and S. Richardson. 1991. The Timed "Up and Go": A test of basic functional mobility for frail elderly persons. *Journal of the American Geriatrics Society* 39:142-148.

Powell, L., and A.M. Myers. 1995. The Activities-specific Balance Confidence (ABC) Scale. *Journal of Gerontology: Medical Sciences* 50A:M28-34.

Raz, I., E. Hauser, and M. Bursztyn. 1994. Moderate exercise improves glucose metabolism in uncontrolled elderly patients with non-insulin-dependent diabetes mellitus. *Israel Journal of Medical Science* 30:766-770.

Rejeski, W.J., L.R. Brawley, W. Ettinger, T. Morgan, and C. Thompson. 1997. Compliance to exercise therapy in older participants with knee osteoarthritis: Implications for treating disability. *Medicine and Science in Sports and Exercise* 29:977-985.

Rejeski, W.J., L.R. Brawley, and S.A. Shumaker. 1996. Physical activity and health-related quality of life. In *Exercise and Sport Sciences Review*, edited by J. Holloszy, 24:71-108.

Richards, T.J., and L. Richards. 1991. The NUD*IST qualitative data analysis system. *Qualitative Sociology* 14:307-324.

Rikkli, R.E., and C.J. Jones. 1997. Assessing physical performance in independent older adults: Issues and guidelines. *Journal of Aging and Physical Activity* 5:244-261.

Rodgers, W.M., and L.R. Brawley. 1991. The role of outcome expectations in participation motivation. *Journal of Sports and Exercise Psychology* 13:411-427.

Roland, M., and R. Morris. 1983. A study of the natural history of back pain, Part I: The development of a reliable and sensitive measure of disability in low back pain. *Spine* 8:141-145.

Rossi, P.H., H.E. Freeman, and M.W. Lipsey. 1999. *Evaluation: A systematic approach*. 6th ed. Thousand Oaks, CA: Sage.

Schneider, J.K. 1996. Qualitative descriptors of exercise in older women. *Journal of Aging and Physical Activity* 4:251-263.

Schneider, S.H., A.K. Khachadurian, L.F. Amorosa, L. Clemow, and N.B. Ruderman. 1992. Ten-year experience with an exercise-based outpatient life-style modification program in the treatment of diabetes mellitus. *Diabetes Care* 15 (Suppl): 1800-1810.

Schnelle, J.F., P.G. MacRae, J.G. Ouslander, S.F. Simmons, and M. Nitta. 1995. Functional inciden-tal training, mobility performance, and incontinence care with nursing home residents. *Journal of the American Geriatrics Society* 43:1356-1362.

Sepsis, P., A. Stewart, B. McLellan, K. Mills, K. Roitz, A. King, and W. Shoumaker. 1995. Seniors' ratings of the helpfulness of health promotion program features in starting and maintaining physical activity. *Journal of Aging and Physical Activity* 3:193-207.

Spink, K.S., and A.V. Carron. 1992. Group cohesion and adherence in exercise class. *Journal of Sport and Exercise Psychology* 14:78-86.

Spirduso, W.W. 1995. *Physical dimensions of aging*. Champaign, IL: Human Kinetics.

Stake, R. 1995. *The art of case study research*. Thousand Oaks, CA: Sage.

Stephens, T. 1988. Physical activity and mental health in the United States and Canada: Evidence from four population surveys. *Preventive Medicine* 17:35-47.

Stephens, T., and C.L. Craig. 1990. *The well-being of Canadians: Highlights of the 1988 Campbell's survey*. Ottawa, ON: Canadian Fitness and Lifestyles Research Institute.

Stewart, A.L., and A.C. King. 1991. Evaluating the efficacy of physical activity for influencing quality of life outcomes in older adults. *Annals of Behavioral Medicine* 13:108-116.

Tinetti, M.E. 1986. Performance-oriented assessment of mobility problems in elderly patients. *Journal of American Geriatrics Society* 34:119-126.

Tinetti, M.E., D. Richman, and L. Powell. 1990. Falls efficacy as a measure of fear of falling. *Journal of Gerontology: Psychological Sciences* 45:P239-P243.

Tudor-Locke, C., and A.M. Myers. 1998. Exercise adoption and maintenance in class-based programs for older men (abstract). *The Gerontologist* 38:170.

Tudor-Locke, C., A.M. Myers, N.W. Rodger, and N.A. Ecclestone. 1998. Towards acceptable exercise guidelines in Type 2 diabetes: An examination of current standards and practices. *Canadian Journal of Diabetes Care* 22:47-53.

United States Department of Health and Human Services. 1992. *Making health communication programs work: A planner's guide*. Washington, DC: U.S. Department of Health and Human Services.

———. 1996. *Physical activity and health: A report of the Surgeon General*. Washington, DC: GPO.

Van Norman, K.A. 1995. *Exercise programming for older adults*. Champaign, IL: Human Kinetics.

Wankel, L.M., and C. Thompson. 1977. Motivating people to be physically active: Self-persuasion vs. balanced decision making. *Journal of Applied Social Psychology* 7:332-340.

Washburn, R.A., K.W. Smith, A.M. Jette, and C.A. Janney. 1993. The Physical Activity Scale for Elderly (PASE): Development and evaluation. *Clinical Journal of Epidemiology* 46:153-162.

Welkowitz, J., R.B. Ewen, and J. Cohen. 1971. *Introductory statistics for the behavioral sciences.* New York: Academic Press.

Wholey, J.S., and K.E. Newcomer. 1997. Clarifying goals, reporting results. *New Directions for Program Evaluation* 75:91-98.

Williams, R.M., and A.M. Myers. 1998a. A new approach to measuring recovery in injured workers with acute low back pain: The Resumption of Activities of Daily Living (RADL) Scale. *Physical Therapy* 78:613-623.

———. 1998b. Functional Abilities Confidence Scale (FACS): A clinically sensible measure for injured workers with acute low back pain. *Physical Therapy* 78:624-634.

Wilson, D., D. Ciliska, J. Singer, K. Williams, J. Alleyne, and E. Lindsay. 1992. Family physicians and exercise counselling: Can they be influenced to provide more? *Canadian Family Physician* 38 (September):2003-2010.

World Health Organization (WHO). 1997. The Heidelberg guidelines for promoting physical activity among older persons. *Journal of Aging and Physical Activity* 5:1-8.

Yin, R.K. 1994. *Case study research: Design and methods.* Thousand Oaks, CA: Sage.

Young Men's Christian Association (YMCA). 1995. *Principles of YMCA health and fitness.* Champaign, IL: Human Kinetics.

Index

About the Author

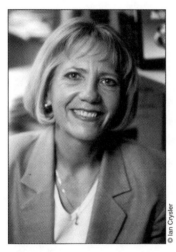

© Ian Crysler

Anita Myers, PhD, is the associate chair of the Department of Health Studies and Gerontology at the University of Waterloo in Waterloo, Ontario. She also is an adjunct professor in the School of Kinesiology at the University of Western Ontario in London, Ontario. She works closely with the Canadian Centre for Activity and Ageing located at the University of Western Ontario in developing and evaluating leadership training and program delivery models.

Myers has also worked with rehabilitation specialists evaluating programs for injured workers and self-management programs for persons with chronic illness. She has directed program evaluations from the grassroots to the national level. Although specializing in exercise programming, she has also conducted broader evaluations of work site health promotion programs. She has published numerous articles, including several outcome measures.

Myers currently serves on the editorial boards of the *Canadian Journal of Program Evaluation* and the *Journal of Aging and Physical Activity*. She is also on the research advisory committee of the Active Living Coalition for Older Adults. She served as chair of professional development and vice president of the Canadian Evaluation Society between 1993 and 1997. In 1997, she received the Contribution to Evaluation in Canada award. She regularly teaches courses in program evaluation at the undergraduate and graduate levels and has delivered over 30 workshops and in-service training seminars on program evaluation to health professions, including exercise leaders and rehabilitation therapists.

Other books from Human Kinetics

Fitness Leader's Handbook

(Second Edition)
B. Don Franks, PhD, and Edward T. Howley, PhD
1998 • Paperback • 272 pp • Item BFRA0654
ISBN 0-88011-654-4 • $24.00 ($35.95 Canadian)

A popular, practical handbook that makes an ideal reference for anyone charged with the task of leading a fitness class.

Health Fitness Management

William C. Grantham, MS, Robert W. Patton, PhD,
Tracy D. York, MS, and Mitchel L. Winick, JD
1998 • Hardcover • 544 pp • Item BGRA0559
ISBN 0-88011-559-9 • $49.00 ($73.50 Canadian)

A comprehensive resource for managing and operating health programs and facilities.

Members for Life

Richard Gerson, PhD
Foreword by John McCarthy
1999 • Paperback • 232 pp • Item BGER0003
ISBN 0-7360-0003-8 • $29.00 ($43.50 Canadian)

Customer service strategies to keep health fitness and sport club members coming back.

To request more information or to order, U.S. customers call 1-800-747-4457, e-mail us at humank@hkusa.com, or visit our website at www.humankinetics.com. Persons outside the U.S. can contact us via our website or use the appropriate telephone number, postal address, or e-mail address shown in the front of this book.

Human Kinetics
The Information Leader in Physical Activity
Code 2335